DENTAL INSTRUMENTS

DENTAL INSTRUMENTS

LORETTA M. CARTER, C.D.A., R.D.A.
Currently in private practice; Formerly Clinical Supervisor,
Dental Auxiliary Utilization Program,
University of Michigan, School of Dentistry,
Ann Arbor, Michigan

PETER YAMAN, B.S., D.D.S., M.S.
Assistant Professor, Department of Operative Dentistry,
University of Michigan, School of Dentistry,
Ann Arbor, Michigan

With assistance from
BETTY LADLEY FINKBEINER, C.D.A., R.D.A., B.S., M.S.

With 553 illustrations

The C. V. Mosby Company
ST. LOUIS • TORONTO • LONDON   1981

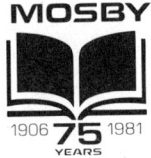

A TRADITION OF PUBLISHING EXCELLENCE

Editor: Darlene A. Warfel
Manuscript editor: Roger McWilliams
Design: Susan Trail
Production: Debbie Wedemeier

Copyright © 1981 by The C.V. Mosby Company

All rights reserved. No part of this book may be reproduced in any manner without written permission of the publisher.

Printed in the United States of America

The C.V. Mosby Company
11830 Westline Industrial Drive, St. Louis, Missouri 63141

Library of Congress Cataloging in Publication Data

Carter, Loretta M
  Dental instruments.

  Bibliography: p.
  Includes index.
  1. Dental instruments and apparatus. I. Yaman, Peter, 1943-   joint author. II. Finkbeiner, Betty Ladley, 1939-   joint author. III. Title.
[DNLM: 1. Dental instruments. WU 26 C324d]
RK681.C37   617.6′0028   80-28707
ISBN 0-8016-0980-1

AC/VH/VH 9 8 7 6 5 4 3 2   01/B/024

CONTRIBUTORS

HENRY E. BRANDAU, B.S., D.D.S., M.S.
Assistant Professor, Department of Operative Dentistry,
University of Michigan, School of Dentistry,
Ann Arbor, Michigan

LORETTA M. CARTER, C.D.A., R.D.A.
Currently in private practice; Formerly Clinical
Supervisor, Dental Auxiliary Utilization Program,
University of Michigan, School of Dentistry,
Ann Arbor, Michigan

FRANK W. COMSTOCK, A.B., D.D.S., M.S.
Professor, Director of Clinics, University of Michigan,
School of Dentistry, Ann Arbor, Michigan

JOHN F. CORCORAN, D.D.S., M.S.
Associate Professor of Dentistry, Chairman,
Department of Endodontics, University of Michigan,
School of Dentistry, Ann Arbor, Michigan

JOHN B. FAUST, B.S., D.D.S., M.S.
Assistant Professor, Department of Orthodontics,
University of Michigan, School of Dentistry,
Ann Arbor, Michigan

BETTY LADLEY FINKBEINER, C.D.A., R.D.A., B.S., M.S.
Instructional Coordinator, Dental Assisting Program,
Washtenaw Community College, Ann Arbor, Michigan

D. JOAN HOLZHAUER, C.D.A., R.D.A.
Senior Dental Assistant, Department of Operative
Dentistry, University of Michigan, School of Dentistry,
Ann Arbor, Michigan

RICHARD A. JOHNSON, B.S., D.D.S., M.S.
Assistant Professor, Department of Orthodontics,
University of Michigan, School of Dentistry,
Ann Arbor, Michigan

CHRISTINE P. KLAUSNER, R.D.H., R.D.A., M.S.
Instructor, Dental Auxiliary Education,
Lansing Community College, Lansing, Michigan

L.H. KLAUSNER, D.D.S., M.S.
Assistant Professor, Department of Operative Dentistry,
University of Michigan, School of Dentistry,
Ann Arbor, Michigan

PAMELA M. PETERS, C.D.A., B.S., M.Ed.
Instructor, Department of Dental Ecology,
University of North Carolina, School of Dentistry,
Chapel Hill, North Carolina

HARVEY SCHIELD, B.S., D.D.S., M.S.
Professor of Dentistry, Preclinical Dentistry,
University of Michigan, School of Dentistry,
Ann Arbor, Michigan

DANIEL T. SNYDER, D.D.S., M.S.
Professor, Department of Operative Dentistry,
University of Michigan, School of Dentistry,
Ann Arbor, Michigan

PETER YAMAN, B.S., D.D.S., M.S.
Assistant Professor, Department of Operative Dentistry,
University of Michigan, School of Dentistry,
Ann Arbor, Michigan

To the late
James B. Bush, D.D.S., M.S.
for his unending dedication and appreciation to
the dental health team

PREFACE

The primary objective of this text is to introduce the dental health team to the physical characteristics, use, and application of instruments necessary to provide dental treatment. The text has been structured according to the six major classifications of dental specialties because of the unique armamentarium of each.

The need exists for a text that consolidates and categorizes dental instruments. We hope that this well-illustrated presentation will facilitate the learning process in this vital area of dental practice.

We would like to express our sincere gratitude to Alayne Spencer-Evans, biomedical illustrator, for her untiring efforts and endless hours in producing quality illustrations for this text.

We are indebted to Isabelle Sands, Joan Holzhauer, Mamie Hall, and Susan McIntyre for providing us with the necessary dental instruments.

We are deeply grateful to Karen Natalie for typing the final manuscript. Her dedication, cooperation, and willingness to help with our project is appreciated.

Loretta M. Carter
Peter Yaman

CONTENTS

1 History of dental instruments, 1
Frank W. Comstock

2 Miscellaneous dental instruments, 4
Betty Ladley Finkbeiner

3 Instruments for isolation, 13
Daniel T. Snyder

4 Hand cutting instruments, 26
Loretta M. Carter

5 Rotary instruments, 39
D. Joan Holzhauer
Peter Yaman

6 Amalgam condensing and cohesive gold instruments, 51
Harvey Schield
Henry E. Brandau

7 Endodontic instruments, 68
John F. Corcoran

8 Orthodontic instruments, 93
John B. Faust
Richard A. Johnson

9 Periodontal instruments, 119
Christine P. Klausner
L.H. Klausner

10 Oral surgery instruments, 147
Pamela M. Peters

11 Instrument sharpening, 165
Christine P. Klausner
L.H. Klausner

12 Instrument sterilization, 175
Loretta M. Carter

Bibliography, 182

1 HISTORY OF DENTAL INSTRUMENTS

Frank W. Comstock

EARLIEST DENTAL INSTRUMENTS

Early in recorded history, dentistry was essentially curative and dealt with the alleviation of pain by assorted palliative methods, including even charms and incantations. Teeth found in skeletons dating as far back as the Neolithic period provide evidence that prehistoric man suffered from dental caries and its attendant pain.[6] There is some evidence that restorative dental procedures were carried out in very early times; excavations in northern Ecuador unearthed skulls of pre-Incans with the teeth filled with gold and cement. The gold was inside of the teeth, and the borings into the tooth structure suggest the use of some sort of "tool."

Probably the first "instruments" used in dentistry were the natural forceps of primitive man—extraction by the finger and thumb. The Greek physician Aristotle (384-322 BC) commented on the extraction of teeth by comparing their removal "by hand" with their removal by "odontagra" (dental forceps). He described dental forceps as being "formed by two levers acting in contrary sense and having a single fulcrum represented by the commissure of the instrument."[6]

It is accurate to assume that, historically, the first dental instruments related to removal of teeth to relieve pain. Galen (200 AD), also a Greek physician, classified teeth and explored their uses. He recognized the nerves of teeth and was the first to propose that the pulp was the sensitive element in teeth. To relieve dental pain, he suggested "the tooth should be perforated with a small trepan (auger) and into the orifices appropriate remedies introduced by means of a director."[6] Reviewing the dentistry of ancient times, one can assume that the earliest rotary instruments were hand-held drills or augers designed to relieve pain and "directors" or carrying instruments to introduce medicines for reducing pain.

The Roman physician Cornelius Celsus (30 BC), who wrote prolifically about the medicine of his period, included detailed descriptions of diseases of the mouth. He described procedures for the extraction of teeth, listing instruments employed in this early dental surgery:

1. Ordinary forceps, for extraction of teeth
2. The rhizagra, for extraction of roots
3. The vulsellum, for removal of splinters
4. The specillum, for exploration, now known as the probe
5. The cautery, a simple, red-hot rod of metal, for application to allay inflammation of gums

Paul of Aegina (7th century), a Roman physician, mentioned the filing of teeth protruding over one another and the smoothing of the sharp edges of broken teeth. "Tartar incrustations," he advised, "should be removed by scrapers or by means of a small file."[6] Certainly this is one of the earliest references to instruments for cleaning teeth. Paul further suggested that hard foods tend to preserve teeth and advised that teeth be cleaned carefully after the last meal of the day.

The fall of the Roman Empire brought a period of stagnation and subsequent retrogression in medicine/dentistry. Rhazes (860-932 AD),[25] an Arabian physician, compared dental caries with caries of the bones and recommended the filling of carious teeth with a compound of mastic and alum called cement. The instruments required for these early efforts of tooth restoration were not described, but one can assume they were crude, limited, and lacking refinement.

MODERN DENTAL INSTRUMENTS

Modern dentistry and dental instruments began to emerge in the 18th century. Pierre Fauchard (1678-1761),[11] the father of modern dentistry, wrote *Les Chirugien dentiste ov traite des dents* in 1728. This was the first comprehensive dental text. In the preface Fauchard speaks of the care that must be taken to keep teeth clean and to fill them. The instruments of Fauchard were hand instruments, crude in comparison to our present equipment. Cavity preparation and the necessary precise instruments were still practically unknown in the 18th century, although instruments for excavating cavities were available and some plastic instruments were developed for placing filling materials.

Our present dental instruments really had their roots in the United States in the 19th century. In 1831 the first adjustable dental chair appeared, followed closely in 1838 by the dental hand drill, patented by John Lewis.[1] J. Foster Flagg's finger- and hand-powered rotary instrument (1846), Chevalier's drill stock (1850), and other inventions were eclipsed in 1871 by Morrison's introduction of the first foot treadle engine. Refinements and improvements on this concept appeared well into the 20th century. Perhaps the most significant contribution to modern restorative dentistry was the introduction and development of the dental electric motor and handpiece by S. S. White from 1870 to 1874. In 1901 the variable-speed (forward and reverse), improved double-lever treadle rheostat dental motor stand was produced. This was refined significantly in 1910 with the introduction of the endless cord on a jointed pulley arm. The angles and handpieces of this era, with speeds of rotation in the 2500- and 5000-rpm range, were precursors of our present low-speed equipment. Contra-angle burs were of the latch type. This belt-and-pulley system continued to be the major power source for dental procedures until the 1950s.

A fascinating source of valuable information about dental instruments and equipment is early dental catalogues.[20,21] Filling materials listed in 1871 include gold foil, tin foil, "composition fillings," and amalgams. A profusion of dental hand instruments is listed: pluggers, condensers, burnishers, scalers, chisels, excavators, burs, and drills. Since Morrison's foot treadle unit had just been introduced in 1871, the burs and drills shown were all applied to restorative problems by hand. Shapes of steel burs included cone, inverted cone, barrel, wheel, round, and "sugarloaf." Bur handles were plain or oc-

HISTORY OF DENTAL INSTRUMENTS

tagonal. Interestingly, rubber dams and rubber dam holders, as well as "rubber dam appliers," were being used by the dental profession more than 100 years ago. A variety of pearl-handled mouth mirrors, pearl-handled lancets and scalers, and cameo-handled instruments with solid-gold ferrules were offered to the dentists of that day.

No review of the history of dental instruments would be complete without mentioning the importance of Dr. G. V. Black's work in organizing, classifying, and identifying dental hand cutting instruments. Black's textbook—*Operative Dentistry, vol. 2*,[4] published in 1908—established for the first time a recognized and accepted classification of the useful forms of excavators, pluggers, and other instruments, along with a nomenclature describing each. Black's instrument formula, using the metric system of measurement, provided an accurate and practical means of instrument description. Blade width, length, and angle were stated in the formula, and when added to the class of the instrument, produced an accurate description. Black's formula and instrument classification are still widely used in dentistry today.

In the last 25 years, the greatest improvement in dental instruments has probably been in the area of rotary equipment. The advent of the diamond point and the tungsten carbide bur, along with ball bearings and the friction-grip chuck, made possible the development of the air turbine and the ultra-high speed of cutting rotation for tooth preparation. With this type of cutting capability in the hands of the skilled practitioner, restorative procedures involving the cutting, shaping, and preparing of enamel and dentin can be carried out with minimum hand pressure, high efficiency, and minimum discomfort to the patient.

Today, dental instruments and equipment in the United States have reached an unsurpassed level of quality and sophistication. Significant improvements in instruments and equipment have contributed greatly to the advent of four-handed dentistry and to the expanding and vital role of the dental auxiliary as active participant in dental patient care. It will be interesting to watch such developments mature in the years ahead.

2 MISCELLANEOUS DENTAL INSTRUMENTS

Betty Ladley Finkbeiner

Some instruments are used for specific procedures in dentistry and may be limited to specialty areas only. Other instruments, however, have multiple uses and may be employed in a variety of situations. The explorer, mirror, and cotton pliers are basic instruments found on most tray setups in a dental office. This chapter provides a review of these and other dental instruments common to many procedures in dentistry.

Explorer

Physical characteristics
1. Single-ended (SE) or double-ended (DE) instrument.
2. Made of steel, with sharp tines, or points.
3. A variety available; the operator's choice often determined by the need to gain access.
4. Fig. 2-1 shows *A*, cowhorn style; *B*, shepherd's hook; *C*, right angle; and *D*, endodontic explorer.

Use

To examine the tooth and detect anomalies through the sense of touch.

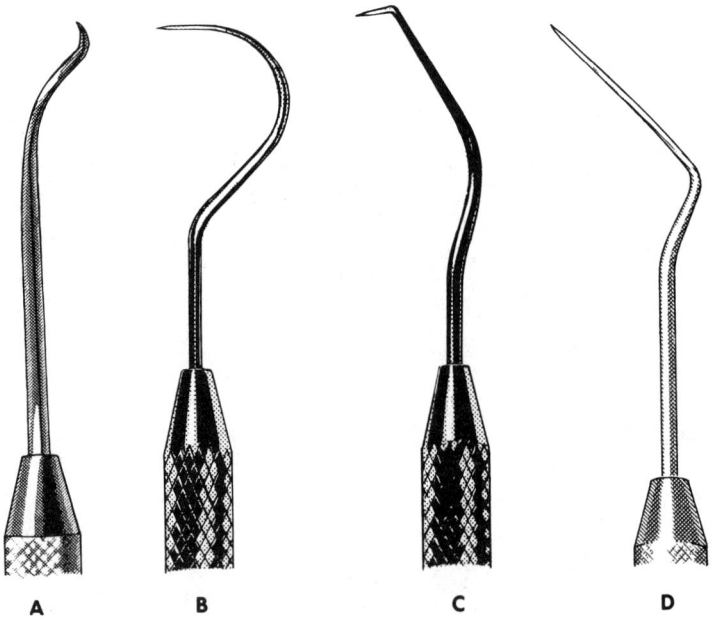

Fig. 2-1

MISCELLANEOUS DENTAL INSTRUMENTS

Mirror

Physical characteristics

1. Range in sizes from ¾ to 1⅝ inches (1.9 to 4 cm).
2. Most detachable, allowing, for example, the mirror attached to a cone-socket stem to be replaced and the handle retained (Fig. 2-2).
3. The face of the mirror is available with a magnifying surface and a plain front surface.
4. In addition to the basic mouth mirror, large mirrors (Fig. 2-3) used for intraoral photography, and hand mirrors used by the patient to check esthetics.

Use

To provide indirect vision, retraction of the lips and cheeks, and illumination of dark areas.

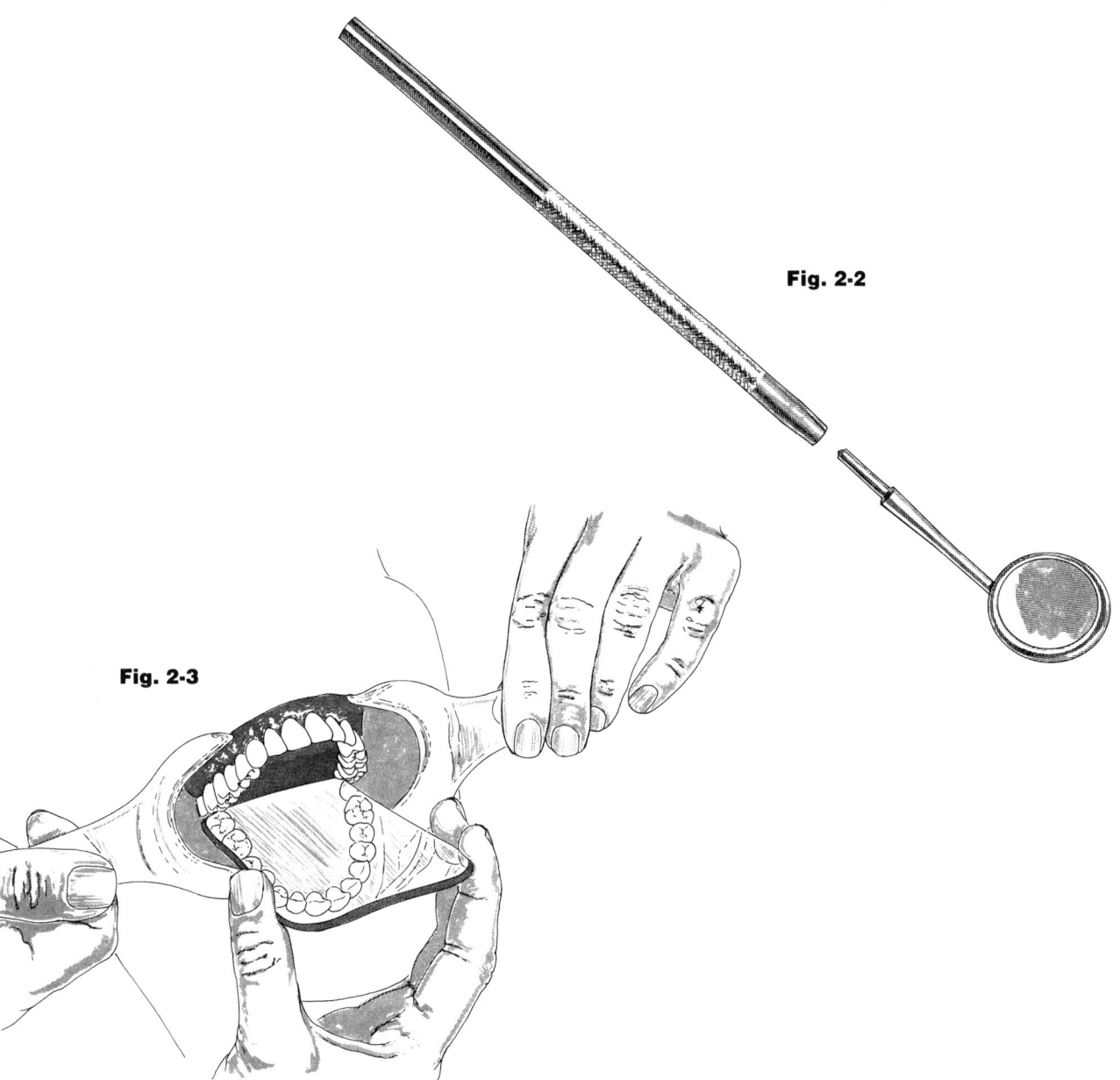

Fig. 2-2

Fig. 2-3

Cotton pliers (forceps)

Physical characteristics
1. Instruments with two blades or beaks and a handle.
2. Various modifications, including locking (Fig. 2-4, *A*) and nonlocking (Fig. 2-4, *B*) pliers.
3. Thumb forceps (Fig. 2-4, *C*) most commonly used to transfer other instruments and materials to and from a tray setup.
4. Articulating paper pliers (Fig. 2-4, *D*) for holding articulating paper in position easily.

Use

To grasp materials or transfer materials in and out of the oral cavity.

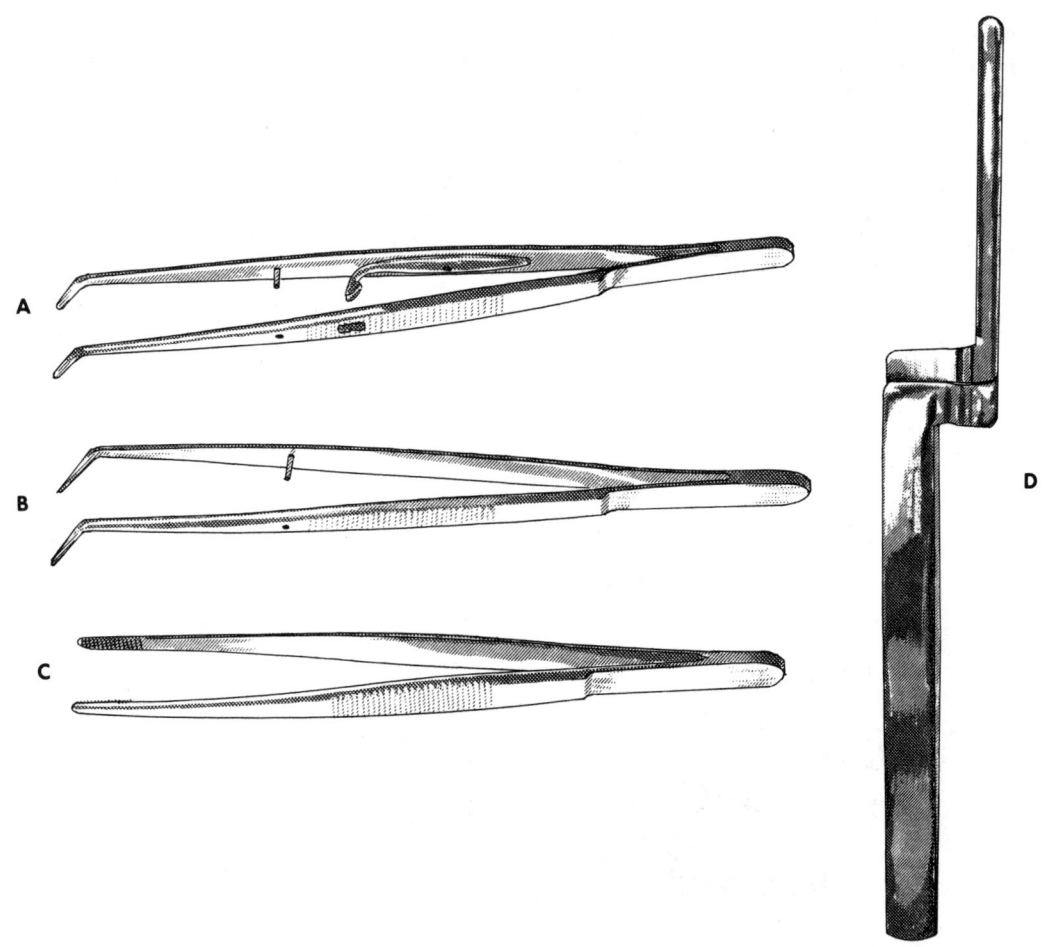

Fig. 2-4

MISCELLANEOUS DENTAL INSTRUMENTS

Dappen dish (Fig. 2-5)

Physical characteristics
1. Small glass or metal dish designed with a large depression at one end and small depression at the other end.
2. Available in several colors to allow color-coding for preprepared tray set-ups.

Use
To hold pastes or liquids, such as polishing paste, disclosing solutions, and powders.

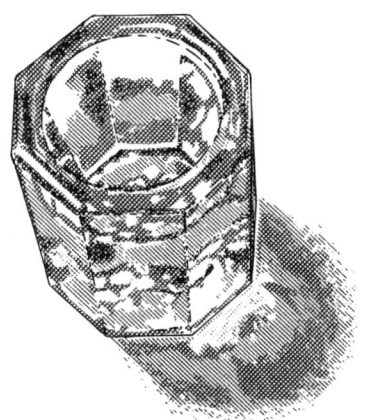

Fig. 2-5

Mixing slabs and pads

Physical characteristics
1. A wide range available.
2. One of the oldest surfaces is a thick, glass slab used to mix common cements (Fig. 2-6).
3. Other mixing surfaces include waxed, nonwaxed, and parchment paper pads (Fig. 2-7).

Use
1. The thick, glass slabs—for mixing zinc phosphate cements.
2. Thin, 2 × 2-inch (5 × 5-cm) glass slabs—for mixing such material as endodontic sealer.
3. Most zinc oxide–eugenol cements mixed on a paper pad, and many manufacturers supply small paper pads on which to mix a cavity liner.

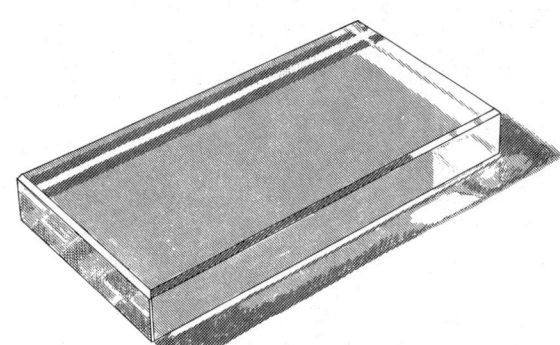

Fig. 2-6

Fig. 2-7

MISCELLANEOUS DENTAL INSTRUMENTS

Spatulas

Physical characteristics
1. Made of plastic (Fig. 2-8, *A*), stainless steel (Fig. 2-8, *B*), or cobalt-chromium alloy (Fig. 2-8, *C*).
2. Usually single-ended instruments with flat, blunt blades either flexible or rigid.
3. Manufacturers provide disposable double-ended spatulas with most restorative materials.

Use

To mix dental cements, liners, impression restoratives, and gypsum materials.

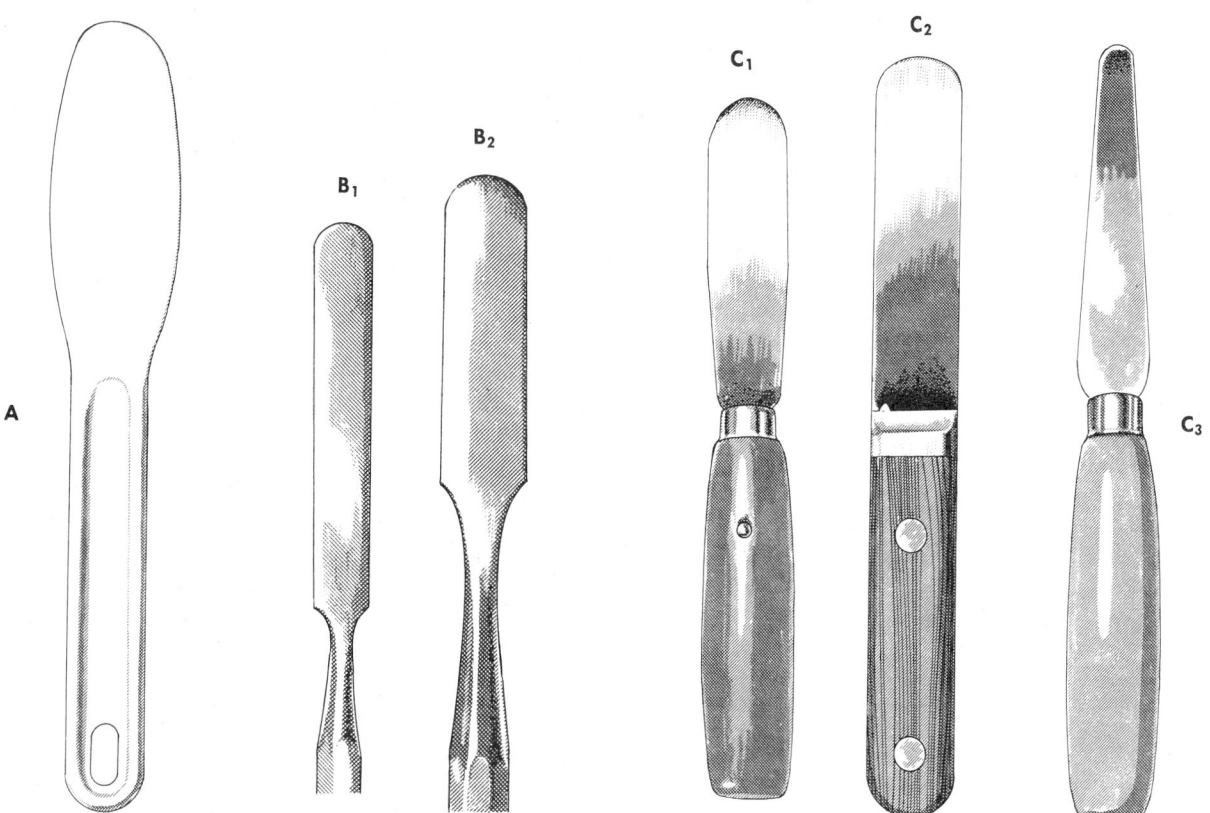

Fig. 2-8

Articulator

Physical characteristics
1. Designed to hold casts of the jaws or teeth in proper alignment during various stages of prosthetic construction.
2. Constructed of metal or plastic in two styles: simple or plain line (Fig. 2-9, *A*) and adjustable (Fig. 2-9, *B*). The simple style provides opening and closing movements on a simple hinge, whereas the adjustable articulator simulates complex jaw movements, such as lateral and protrusive thrust.
3. Available in a quadrant, simple full arch, or a more complicated full arch.

Use
1. A simple articulator may be used in the processing of inlays, crowns, and bridges.
2. During denture construction a more complicated articulator is necessary to duplicate jaw movement.

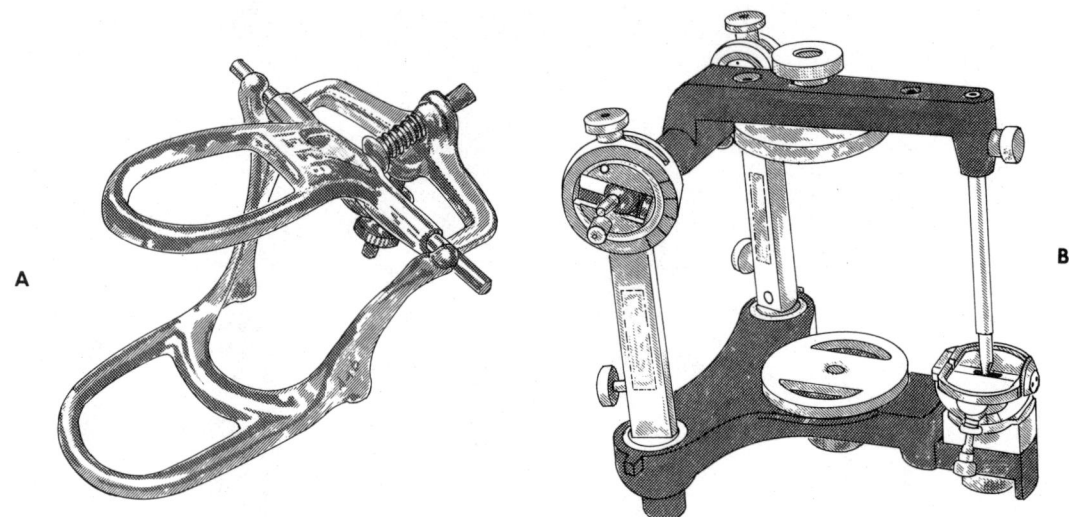

Fig. 2-9

MISCELLANEOUS DENTAL INSTRUMENTS

Mouth props Physical characteristics
1. Made of rubber, with a serrated edge on which the maxillary and mandibular teeth may rest while the mouth remains open (Fig. 2-10).
2. Molt mouth prop (Fig. 2-11) similar to rubber mouth prop but with characteristics of a hemostat to vary the degree of opening.

Use

To assure the mouth remains open during prolonged treatment; placed in the mouth with the narrow portion toward the distal.

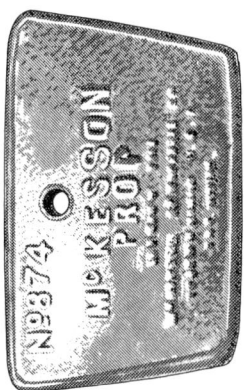 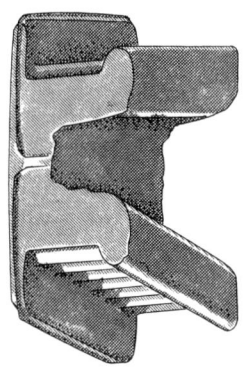

Fig. 2-10

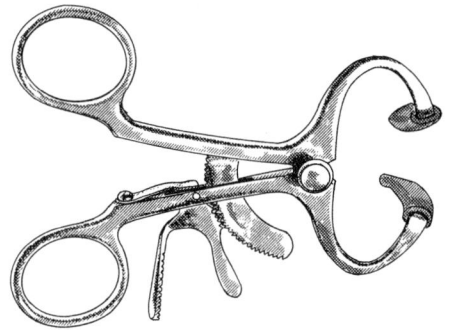

Fig. 2-11

Bachus towel clamp
(Fig. 2-12)

Physical characteristics
Hemostat-like instrument with beaks resembling a cowhorn configuration.

Use
1. Normally for surgical use.
2. Modified to grasp materials, such as removing aluminum shell crowns from the mouth by placing the beaks on the buccal and lingual aspects and lifting in an occlusal direction.

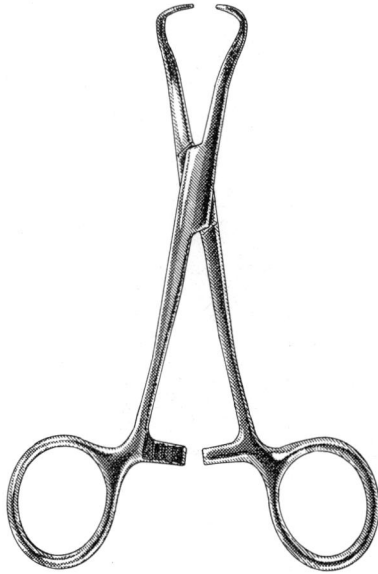

Fig. 2-12

3 INSTRUMENTS FOR ISOLATION

Daniel T. Snyder

Quality restorative dentistry treatment is best performed when there is adequate control of the oral operating field. Biomechanical principles can be used more effectively in cavity preparation when conditions provide optimum vision, removal of moisture, and access for instrumentation to ensure proper manipulation and insertion of restorative materials.

Several methods may be employed to accomplish an adequate operating field. Primary control of the field consists of isolating the involved tooth and its quadrant from oral fluids and the tongue, cheek, and lips. Adjunctive instruments and devices for the removal of moisture and debris are also important to the maintenance of the operative field.

This chapter will describe and illustrate the materials, instruments, and devices that effectively control the operating field for restorative dentistry.

Rubber dam

Physical characteristics
1. A thin, pliable rubber material, cut in 5- and 6-inch (12.5- and 15-cm) squares.
2. Available in medium, heavy, extra-heavy, or special-heavy thickness and light or dark shades.

Use
To isolate teeth from the surrounding oral environment (Fig. 3-1).

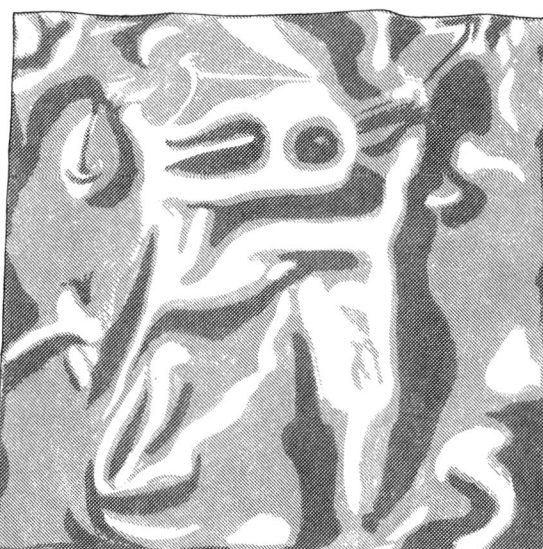

Fig. 3-1

Rubber dam frame

Physical characteristics
1. Available in a plastic circular form with peripheral projections (Fig. 3-2, *A*).
2. Metal frames U shaped, 4 × 4 inches (10 × 10 cm), with projections on which the rubber dam is retained (Fig. 3-2, *B*).
3. Strap style composed of two metal pieces with spring clips joined by cloth straps surrounding the patient's neck to provide tension to retain the rubber dam in place (Fig. 3-2, *C*).

Use
To retain and stabilize the rubber dam during application.

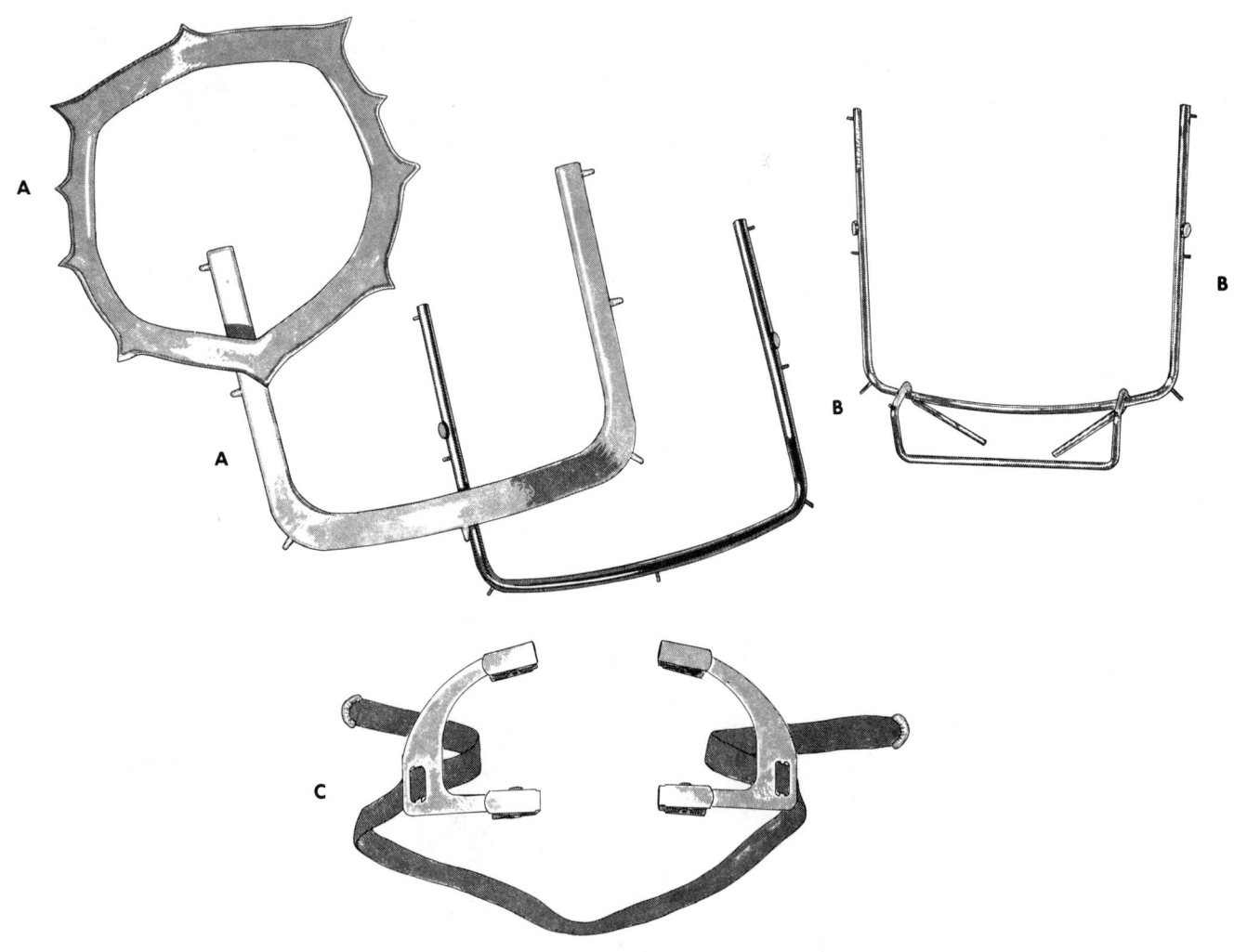

Fig. 3-2

INSTRUMENTS FOR ISOLATION

Rubber dam clamps
(Fig. 3-3)

Physical characteristics
1. Available in winged (Fig. 3-3, *A*) and wingless (Fig. 3-3, *B*) styles.
2. Fabricated with stainless steel or chrome-plated steel.
3. Jaws joined by the bow portion that is expanded with forceps during placement on the tooth.

Use
To retain and retract the rubber dam on the tooth to which it is applied.

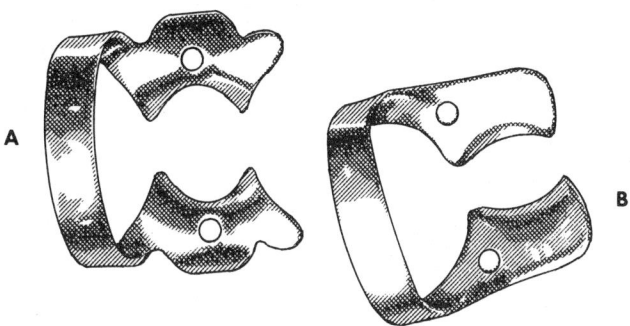

Fig. 3-3

Rubber dam punch
(Fig. 3-4)

Physical characteristics
1. Plierslike instrument.
2. Working end contains a punch device on one side and a rotating table, with six different-sized holes, on the other side.

Use
To punch holes of appropriate size in the rubber dam material.

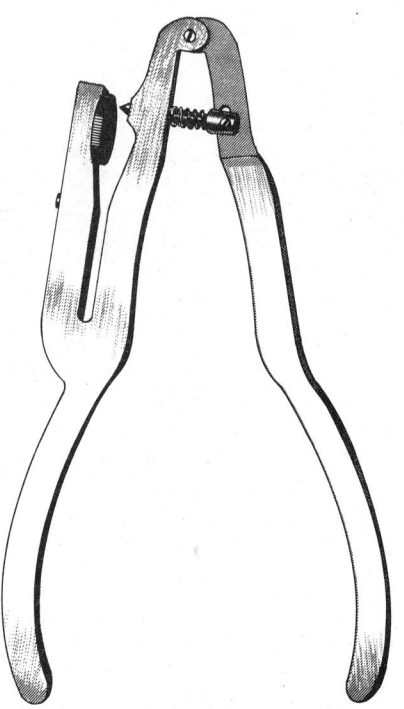

Fig. 3-4

INSTRUMENTS FOR ISOLATION

Rubber dam forceps
(Fig. 3-5)

Physical characteristics
1. Plierslike forceps.
2. When squeezed, the handles open the working end.
3. Beaklike projections on the tip of the working end insert into the rubber dam clamp holes.

Use
To expand the rubber dam clamp for insertion around the tooth.

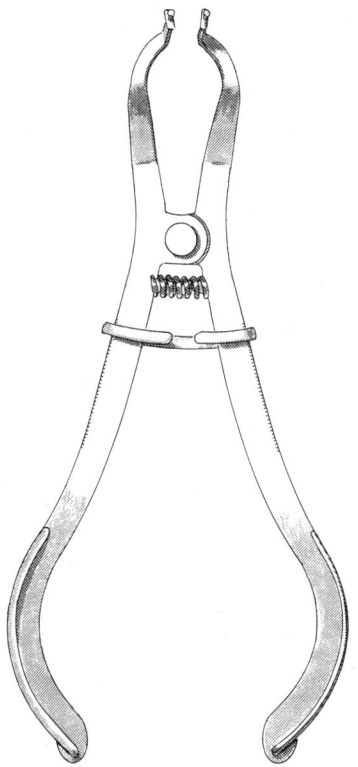

Fig. 3-5

Ligatures

Physical characteristics
Available as waxed dental floss.

Use
1. Tied around a tooth to retain and retract the rubber dam when a clamp is not feasible.
2. To aid in the passage of the rubber dam through the interdental contacts.

Rubber dam gauze mask
(Fig. 3-6)

Physical characteristics
1. Fabricated in cotton gauze material.
2. Available to match the rubber dam size.
3. Shaped with a central cutout for the oral cavity.

Use
To be placed between the patient's face and the rubber dam for comfort.

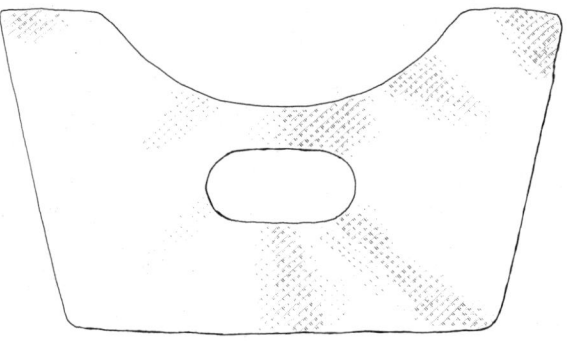

Fig. 3-6

INSTRUMENTS FOR ISOLATION

Straight scissors (Fig. 3-7)

Physical characteristics
1. Made of chrome-plated metal.
2. Slender, 4¾ inches (11.9 cm) long.

Use

To cut the interseptal portion of the rubber dam during its removal.

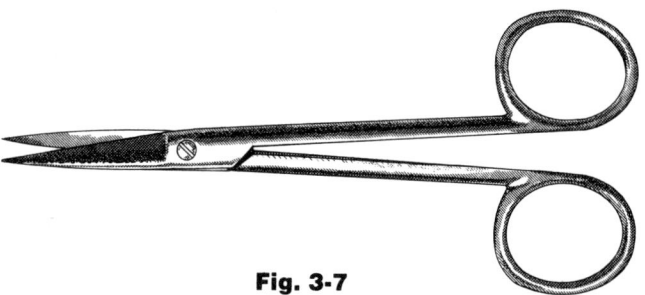

Fig. 3-7

Rubber dam

Application

Fig. 3-8.

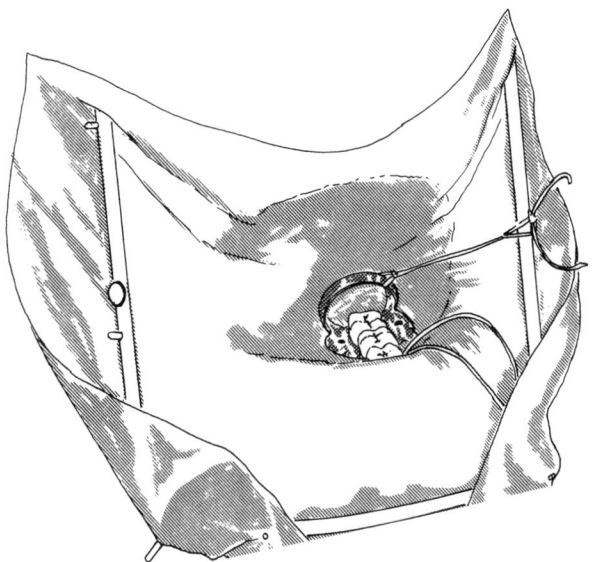

Fig. 3-8

19

Cotton rolls (Fig. 3-9)

Physical characteristics
1. Made of cylindrical, compressed cotton fibers with a diameter of ⅜ to ½ inch (0.9 to 1.3 cm).
2. Fabricated in lengths of 1½, 2, 2½, and 6 inches (3.8, 5, 6.3, and 15 cm).
3. Available with quilted covering.

Use
To isolate teeth from the oral environment when rubber dam application is not feasible.

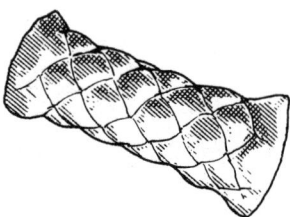 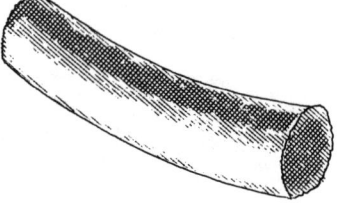

Fig. 3-9

INSTRUMENTS FOR ISOLATION

Cotton roll holders (Fig. 3-10)

Physical characteristics
1. Plated metal construction.
2. Available in child and adult sizes.
3. Spoon-shaped holder fits under the patient's chin (Fig. 3-10, *B*).

Use

To accept the attachment of cotton rolls; positioned around the buccal and lingual aspects of a quadrant of mandibular teeth (Fig. 3-10, *A*).

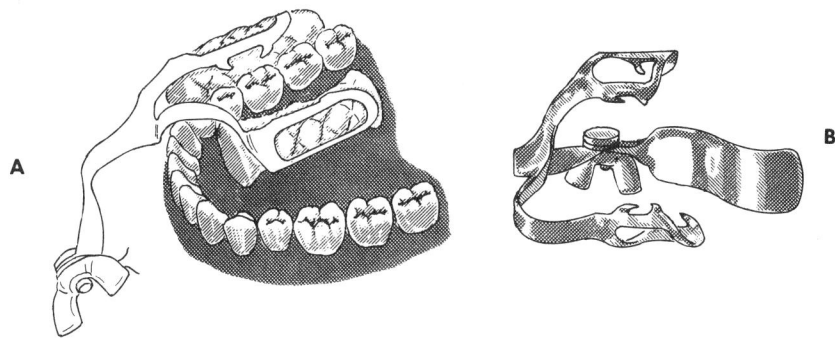

Fig. 3-10

Absorbent wafer (Fig. 3-11)

Physical characteristics
1. Triangular shaped.
2. Available in small and large sizes with sides 1½ or 1¾ inches (3.8 or 4.4 cm) long.
3. Fabricated of compressed paper wafer, with foil on one side (Fig. 3-11).

Use

To control salivary flow when placed adjacent to the parotid opening in the maxillary vestibule.

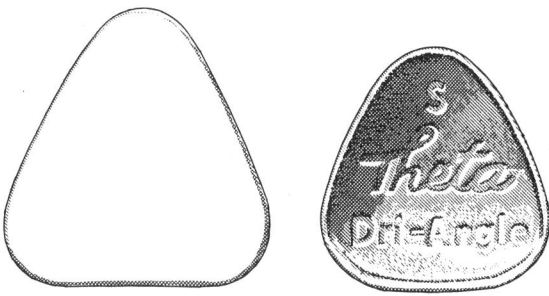

Fig. 3-11

Saliva ejector

Physical characteristics
1. Tubular-shaped, with a ¼-inch (0.6-cm) diameter (Fig. 3-12, *A* and *B*).
2. Available in metal or plastic.
3. Metal type (svedopter) available with three tongue retraction plates in 1¼- to 1⅞-inch (3.2- to 4.8-cm) widths (Fig. 3-12, C_1).
4. The plastic type formed as desired (Fig. 3-12, *A*).

Use
To evacuate reduced volumes of fluids from the oral cavity (Fig. 3-12, *B*, C_2, and D_1).

INSTRUMENTS FOR ISOLATION

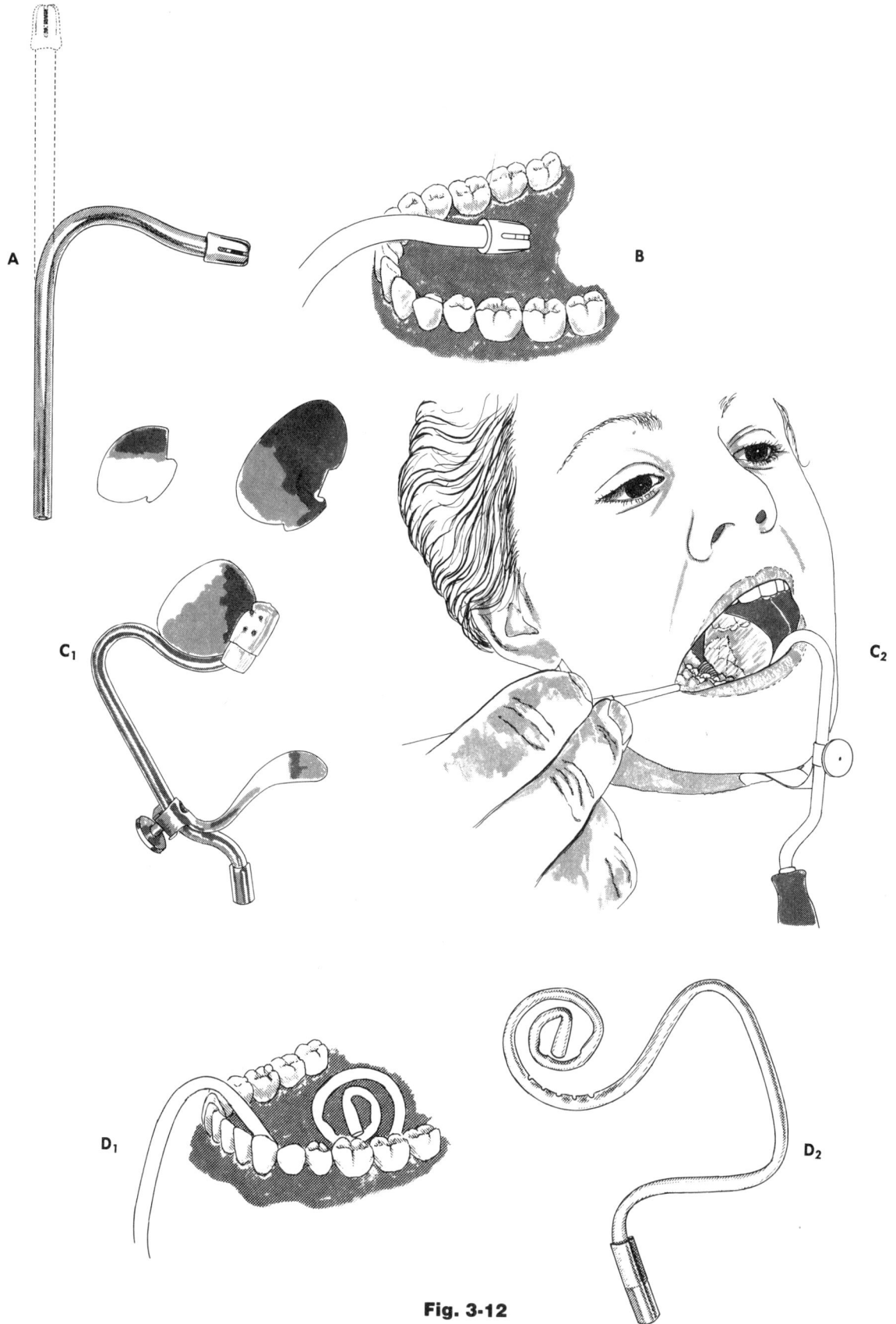

Fig. 3-12

High-volume evacuator (HVE)

Physical characteristics
1. Available in various sizes and shapes.
2. Disposable, plastic type tubular-shaped and straight, with a 7/16-inch (1.1 cm) diameter and a 4½-inch (11.3-cm) length (Fig. 3-13, *A*).
3. Plastic and metal reusable types tubular-shaped, curved or angled, and 6 to 7 inches (15 to 17.5 cm) in length (Fig. 3-13, *B* and *C*).
4. May have beveled ends.
5. May also have attached plate- or spoon-shaped end-piece (Fig. 3-13, *D*).
6. Vacuum-ejector system with bite blocks and specialized tongue retractor components (Fig. 3-13, *E*).

Use
To evacuate large volumes of fluids and debris from the oral cavity.

Application
Fig. 3-14.

INSTRUMENTS FOR ISOLATION

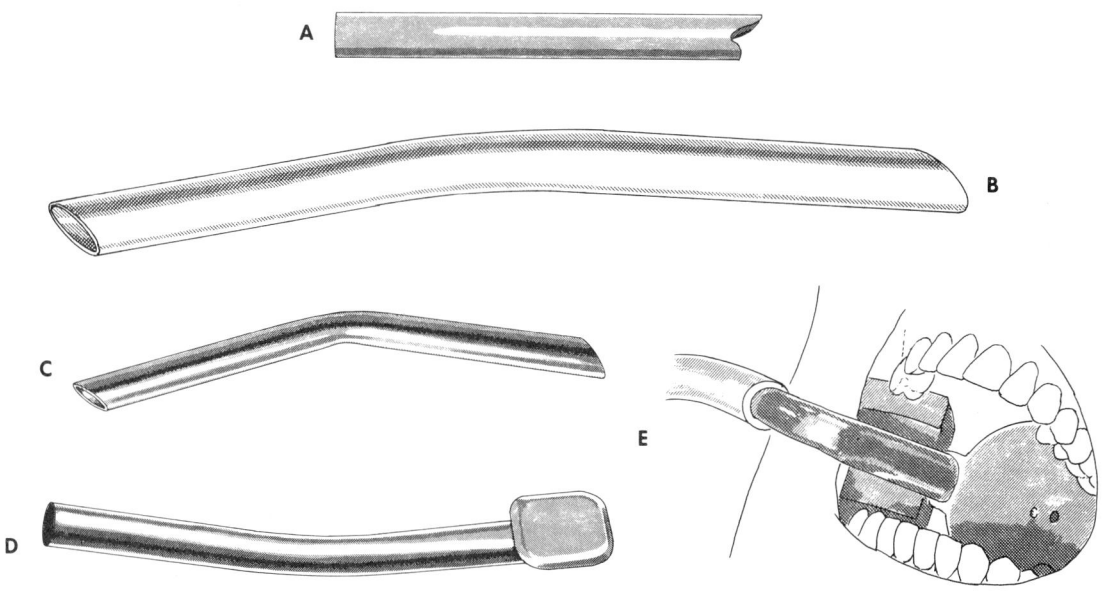

Fig. 3-13

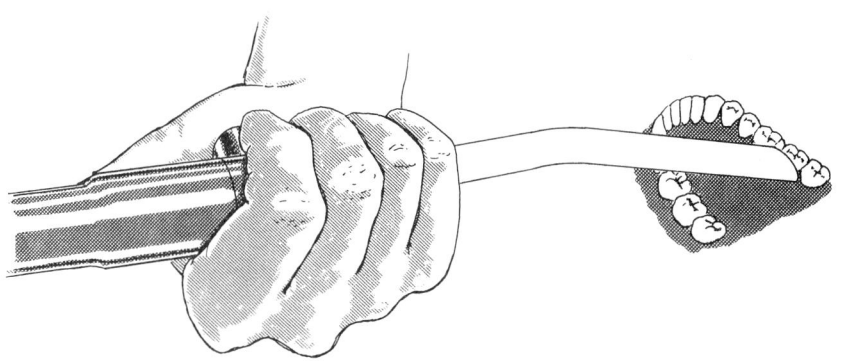

Fig. 3-14

4 HAND CUTTING INSTRUMENTS

Loretta M. Carter

Hand cutting instruments were designed to help in the preparation of cavity restoration. To properly use hand cutting instruments, it is necessary to learn the basic design and the function of each.

G. V. Black developed a standardized nomenclature for dental instruments that provides classifications and categories. This nomenclature aids in the regulation of dental instrument design. The three basic parts of a hand cutting instrument include (Fig. 4-1, *A*):

1. *Blade,* or *nib*—the functional end of the hand instrument, containing the cutting edge or condenser.
2. *Shank*—"connector" between the handle and blade; it may be single-, double-, or triple-angled or have no angle.
3. *Handle,* or *shaft*—the portion of the hand instrument held by the operator; it may be serrated, knurled, or smooth.

The G. V. Black formula is a simple, functional, three-unit formula used to describe the design of the basic dental instrument. The formula consists of the following units (Fig. 4-1, *B*):

1. The width of the blade measured in tenths of millimeters.
2. The length of the blade measured in millimeters.
3. The angle the blade forms with the long axis of the handle in centigrades (100 degrees for complete circle).

HAND CUTTING INSTRUMENTS

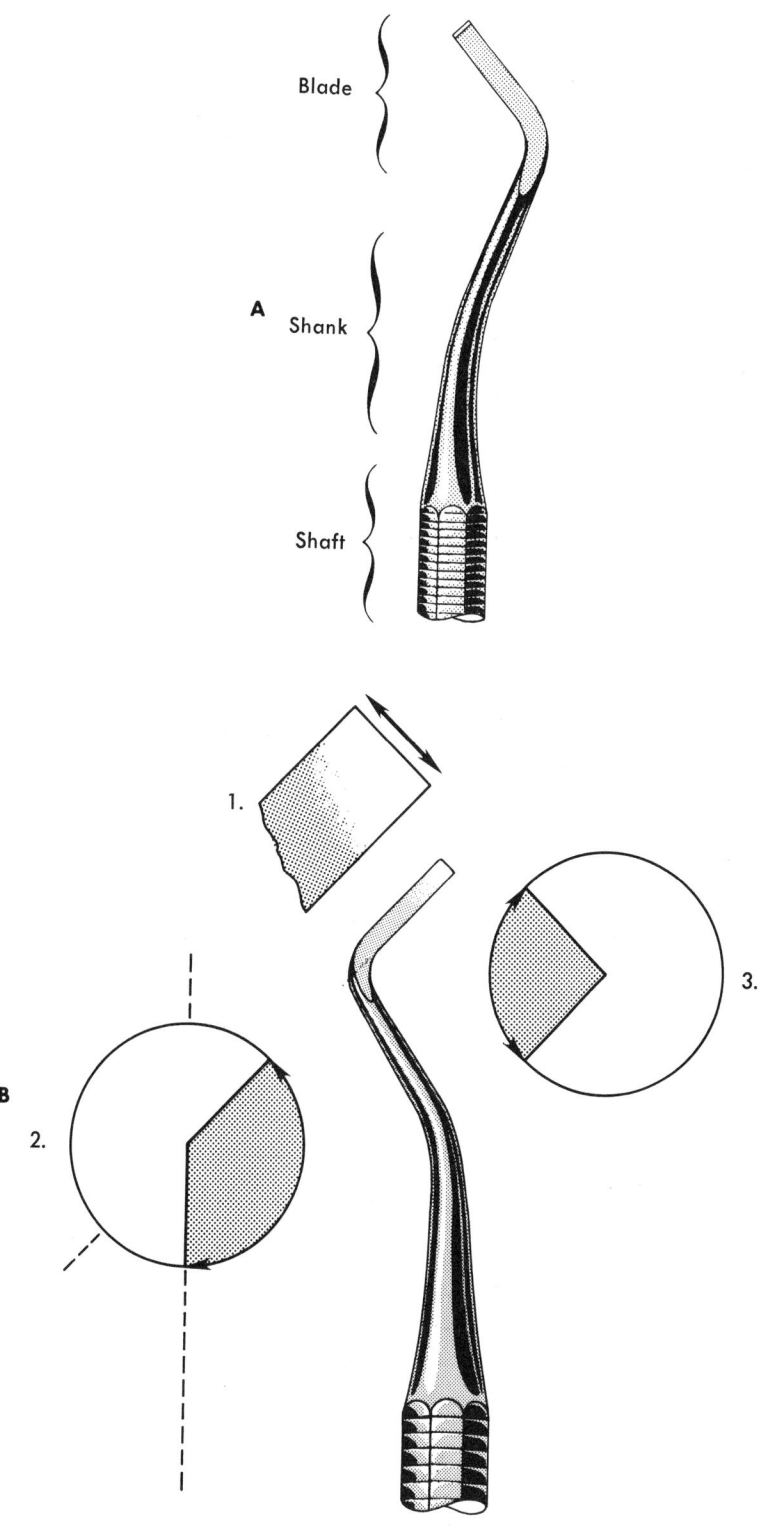

Fig. 4-1

This formula is utilized with all dental hand instruments. Hand cutting instruments will vary in the number of angles the shank will take to the long axis of the handle. Examples of different angles are:
1. Straight—shank containing no angle (Fig. 4-2).
2. Monangle—shank containing one angle (Fig. 4-3).
3. Biangle—shank containing two angles (Fig. 4-4).
4. Triple angle—shank containing three angles (Fig. 4-5).

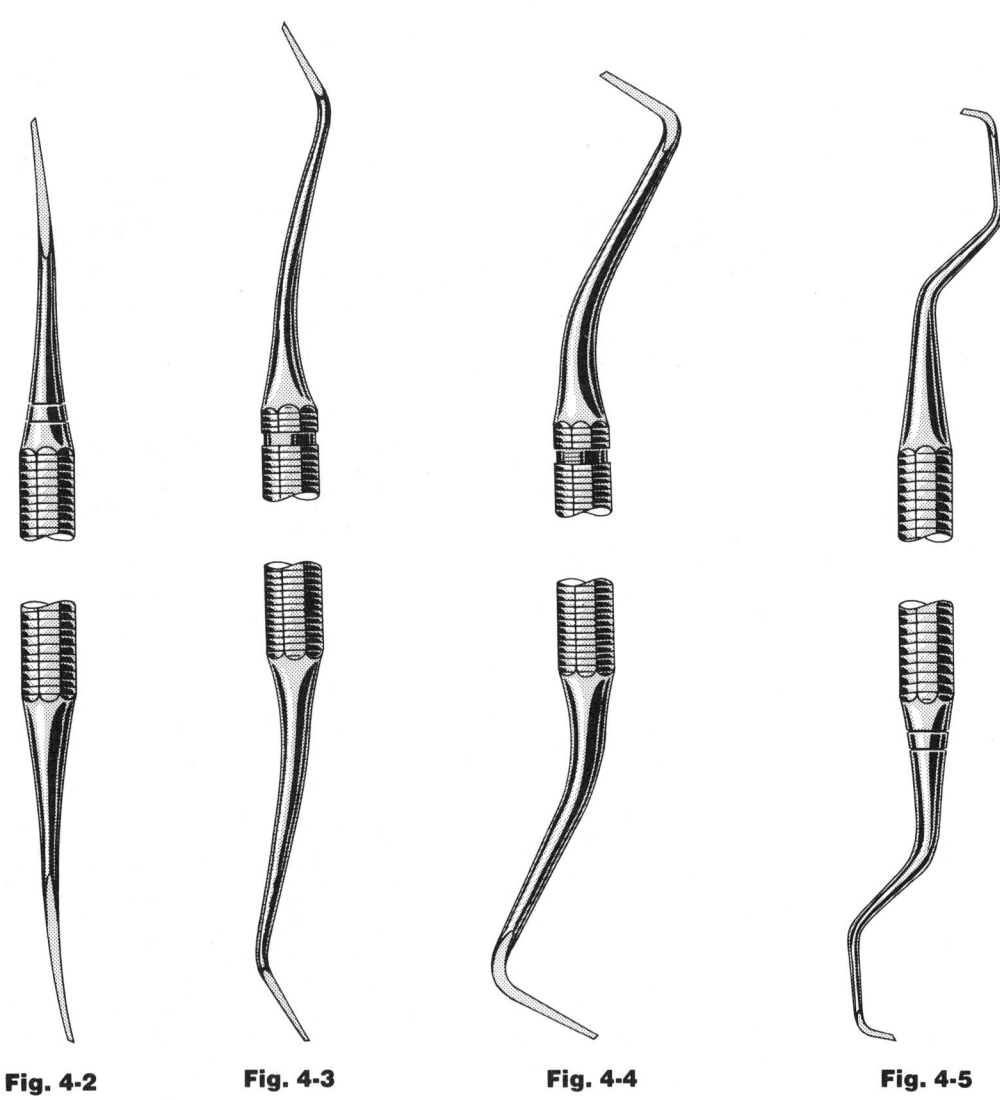

Fig. 4-2   Fig. 4-3   Fig. 4-4   Fig. 4-5

HAND CUTTING INSTRUMENTS

CHISELS The cutting edge of a chisel forms a right angle with the long axis of the handle. When these instruments are double-ended, one cutting edge is distal to the handle and is termed "reverse bevel" (Fig. 4-6, *A*). The other end is the "standard bevel" (Fig. 4-6, *B*). The reverse bevel is indicated on the instrument shaft by an indented ring.

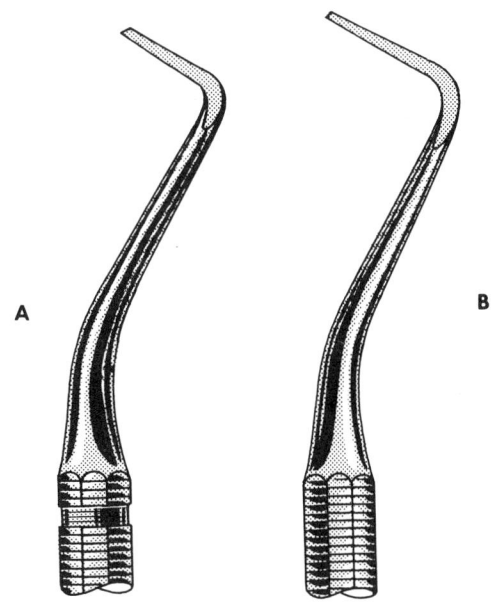

Fig. 4-6

Straight chisel (Fig. 4-7, A)

Physical characteristics
1. Straight-angle instrument with a one-sided bevel.
2. Double-ended instrument.
3. Cutting edge at right angle with long axis of handle.

Use
For planing and cleaving enamel.

Application
Because of its design, primarily used in the maxillary arch with a palm grasp (Fig. 4-7, B).

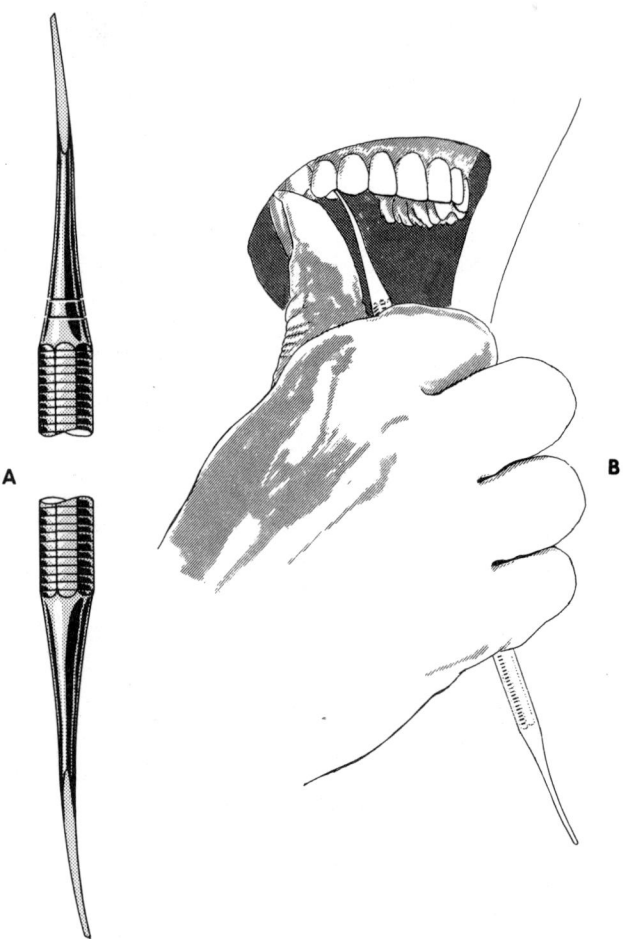

Fig. 4-7

HAND CUTTING INSTRUMENTS

Monangle chisel
(Fig. 4-8, A)

Physical characteristics
1. Monangle instrument with a triple cutting surface.
2. Double-ended instrument, designed with a right *(R)* and left *(L)* of the instrument cutting edge.

Use
To define line and point angles of a cavity preparation.

Application
Fig. 4-8, *B*.

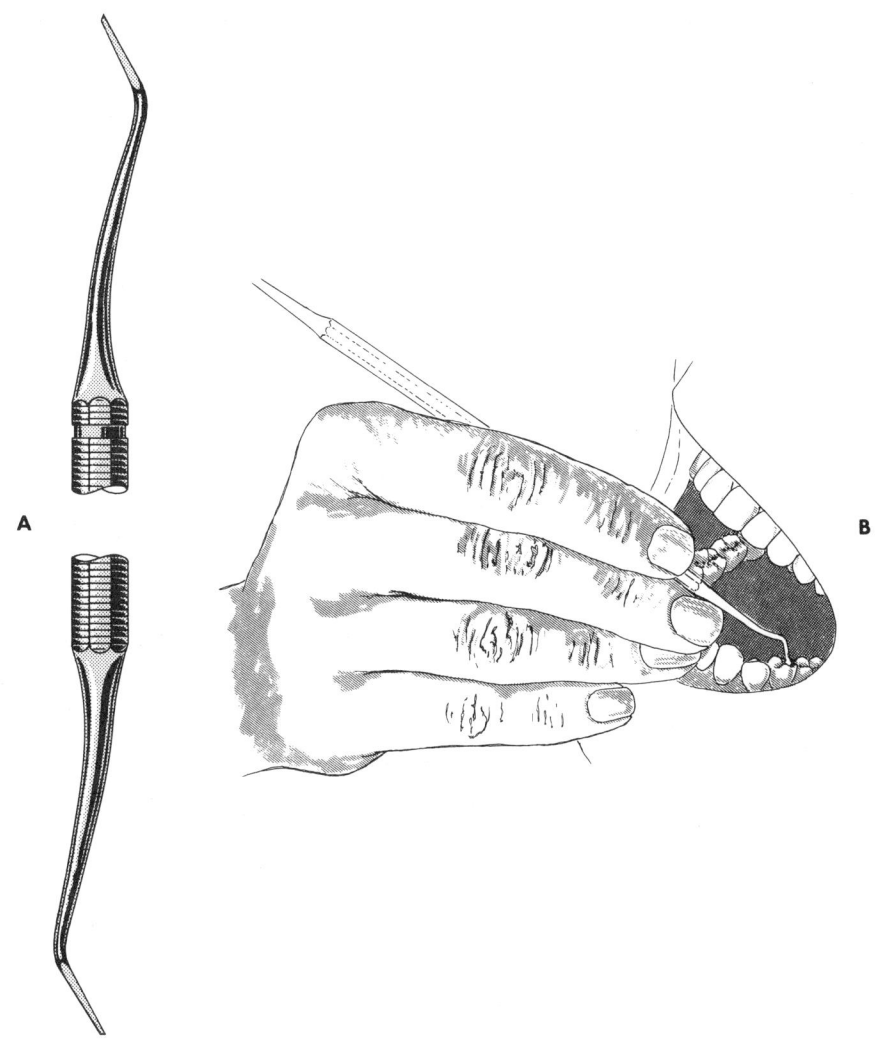

Fig. 4-8

Biangle chisel (Fig. 4-9, A)

Physical characteristics
1. Two angles in the shank and shaft of instrument for accessibility.
2. Double-ended instrument, with a reverse and standard bevel indicated by indented ring on handle.

Use
To remove enamel rods from floor of cavity with a push action.

Application
Fig. 4-9, B.

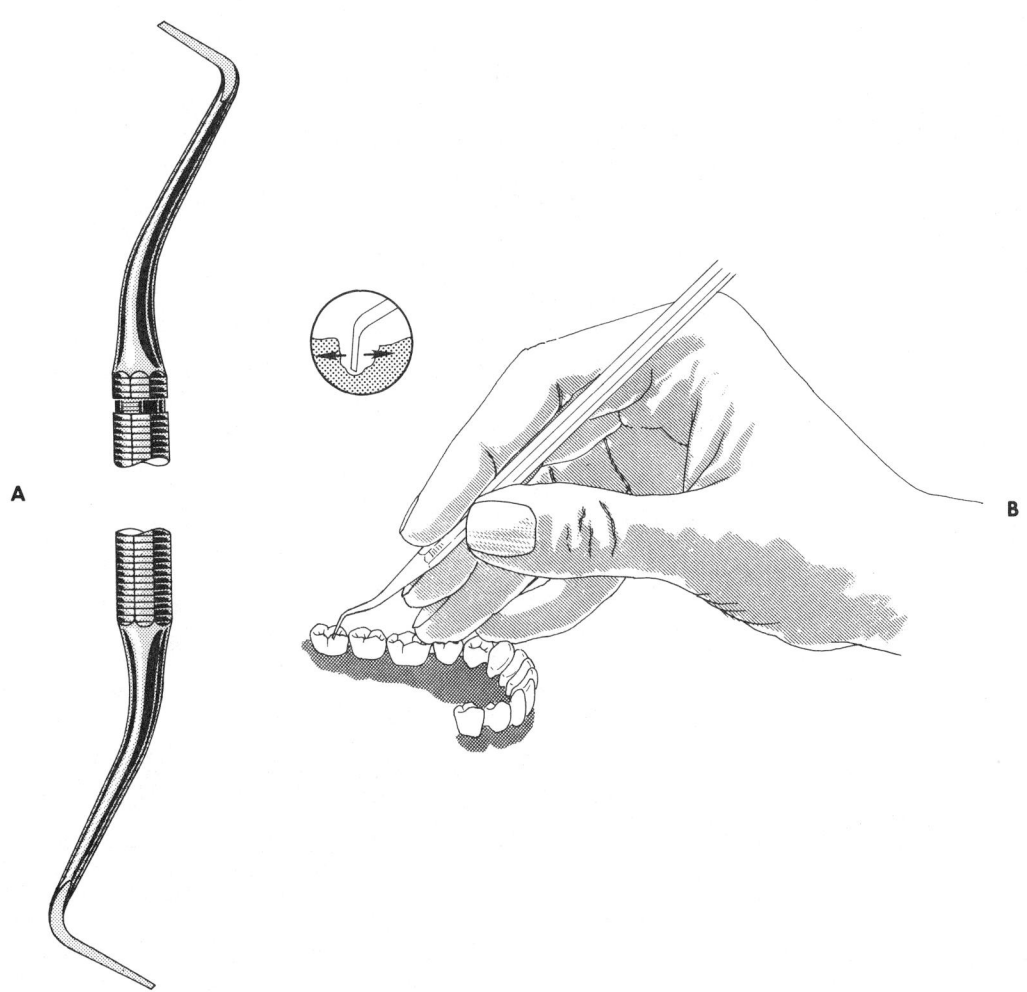

Fig. 4-9

HAND CUTTING INSTRUMENTS

Triple-angle chisel
(Fig. 4-10, A)

Physical characteristics
1. A modification of a chisel, called a *hoe*. The instrument with a blade angulation greater than 12.5 centigrades considered to be a hoe.
2. Reverse and standard bevel indicated on the handle by the indented ring.

Use
For planing and cleaving of enamel with a pull action.

Application
Fig. 4-10, *B*.

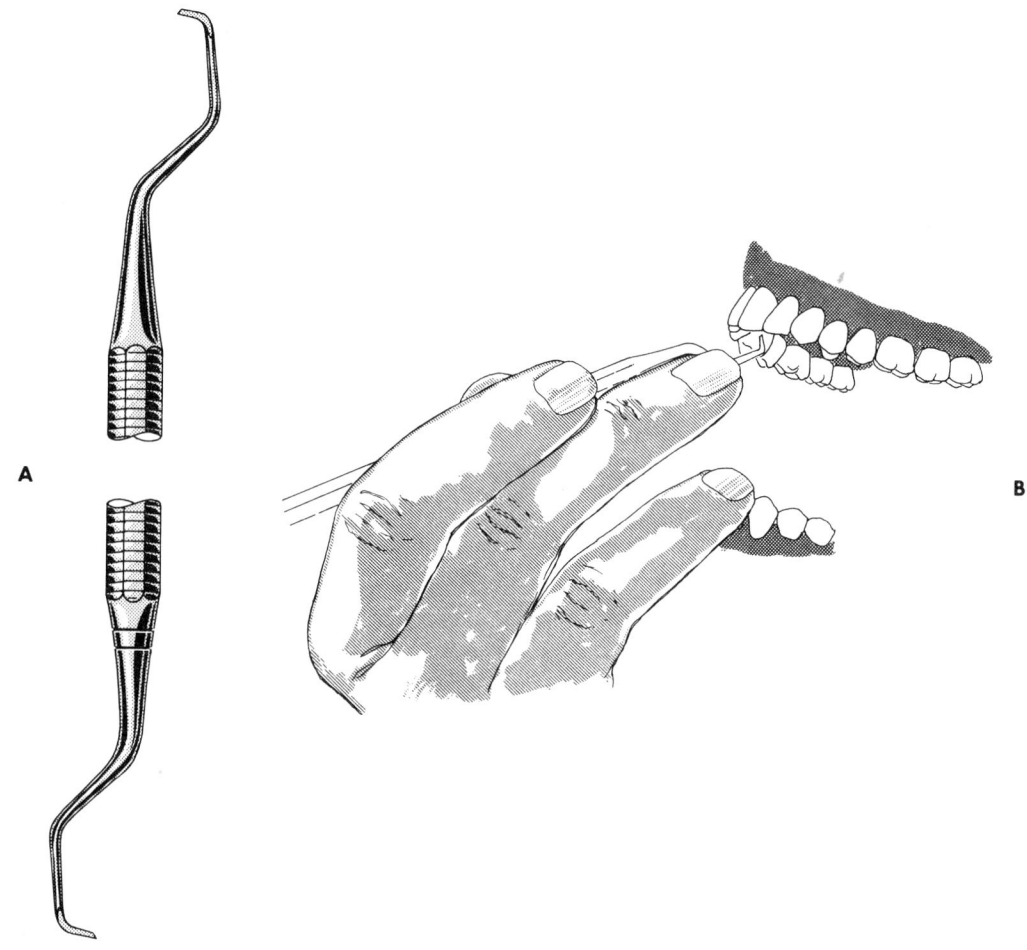

Fig. 4-10

Biangle-angle chisels
(Fig. 4-11)

Physical characteristics
1. Modification of the enamel chisel.
2. Contains triple cutting surface.

Use
To remove enamel from cavity walls.

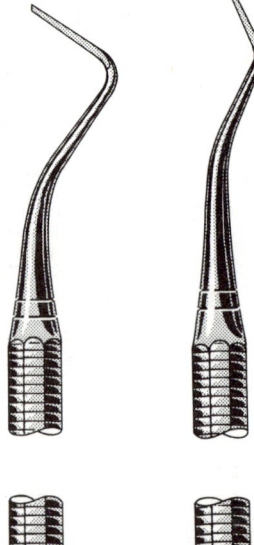

Fig. 4-11

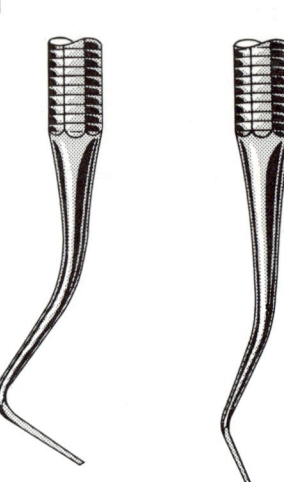

HATCHETS The cutting edge of an enamel hatchet is parallel to the angle of the handle of an instrument. Consequently, enamel hatchets will have a *right* and *left* of an instrument or a pair of instruments. With the instrument in working position, the bevel to the right of the blade will be the *left* cutting edge and the bevel to the left will be the *right* cutting edge. The right and left of a pair will be indicated by the indented ring on the handle.

Basic enamel hatchet
(Fig. 4-12, *A*)

Physical characteristics
1. Biangle instrument with cutting edge parallel to long axis of handle.
2. Right *(R)* and left *(L)* of an instrument; indented ring indicates *R* of pair (Fig. 4-12, *B*).
3. Designed to come in pairs, with a large and a small pair.

Use
Primarily to obtain retention form in a cavity preparation and to cleave enamel from cavity walls.

Application
Fig. 4-12, *C*.

HAND CUTTING INSTRUMENTS

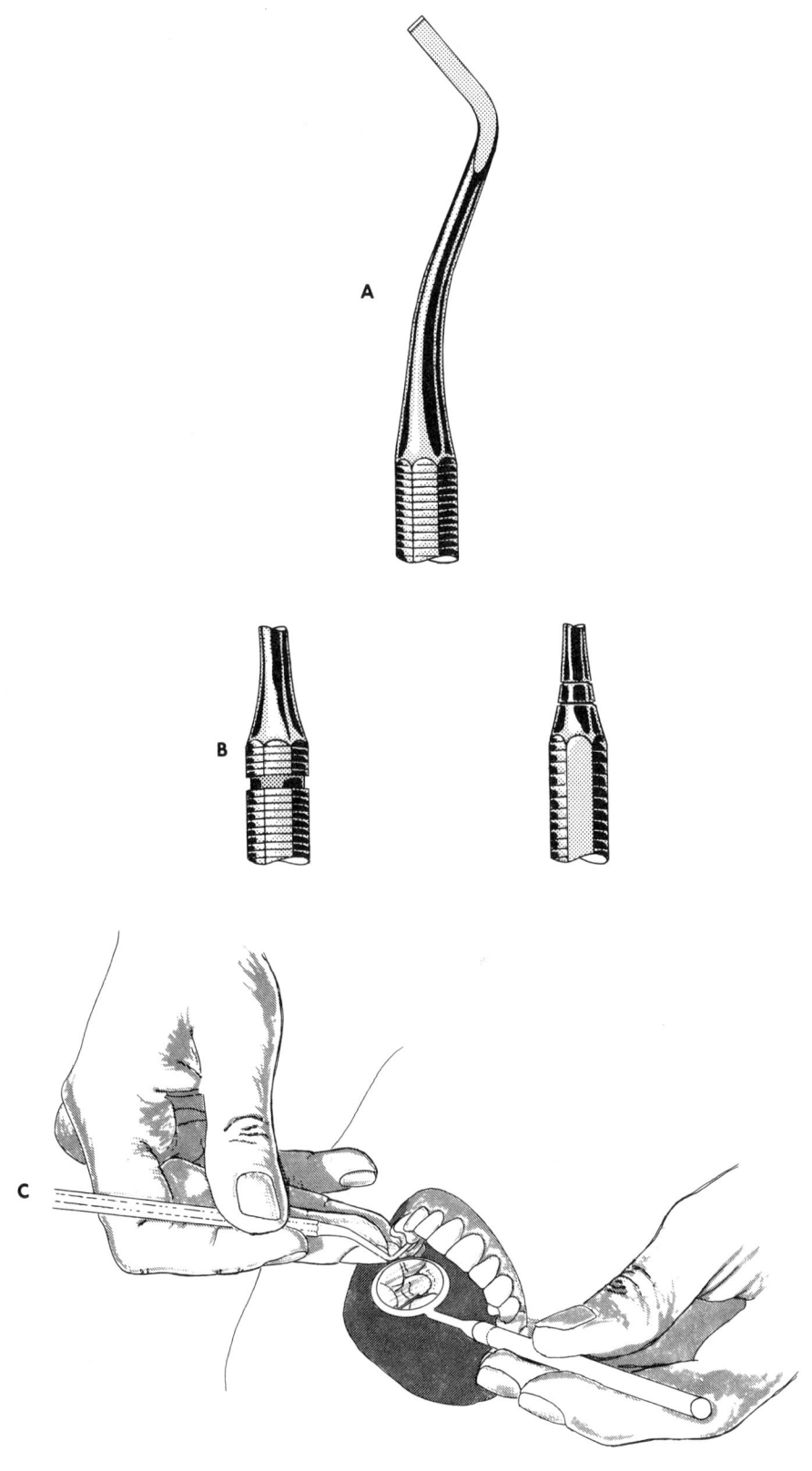

Fig. 4-12

Gingival margin trimmers

Physical characteristics
1. Modification of an enamel hatchet.
2. Double-planed instrument.
3. Curved blade, forming another angle, as opposed to the straight blade of the basic enamel hatchet (Fig. 4-13, *A*).
4. Contains four numbers in the G. V. Black formula for hand cutting instruments to give the second angle of the blade a number, for example, 10-95-6-12. The second number indicates the angle the cutting edge takes to the long axis of the handle in centigrades.
5. Small (Fig. 4-13, *B*) and large trimmers (Fig. 4-13, *C*).

Use
1. To bevel the cervical walls of the distal-proximal and mesial-proximal of an inlay preparation.
2. To remove unsupported enamel from the cervical floor of amalgam preparation.

Application
Fig. 4-13, *D*.

HAND CUTTING INSTRUMENTS

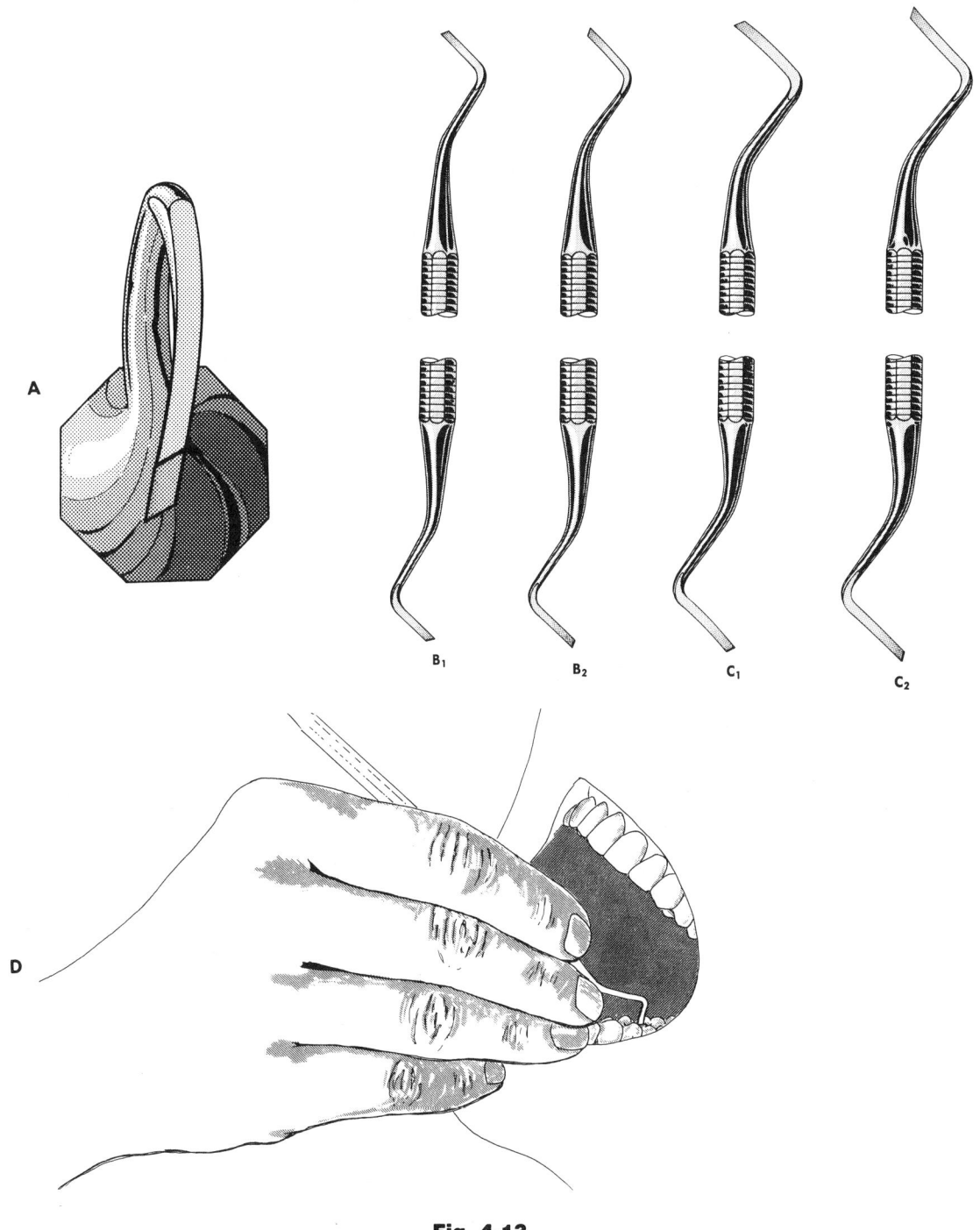

Fig. 4-13

Spoon excavator
(Fig. 4-14, A)

Physical characteristics
1. Spoon shaped.
2. Biangle instrument.
3. Entire cutting edge sharpened.
4. Modified hatchet; cutting edge parallel to long axis of handle.

Use
Cutting surface designed to remove carious dentin.

Application
Fig. 4-14, B.

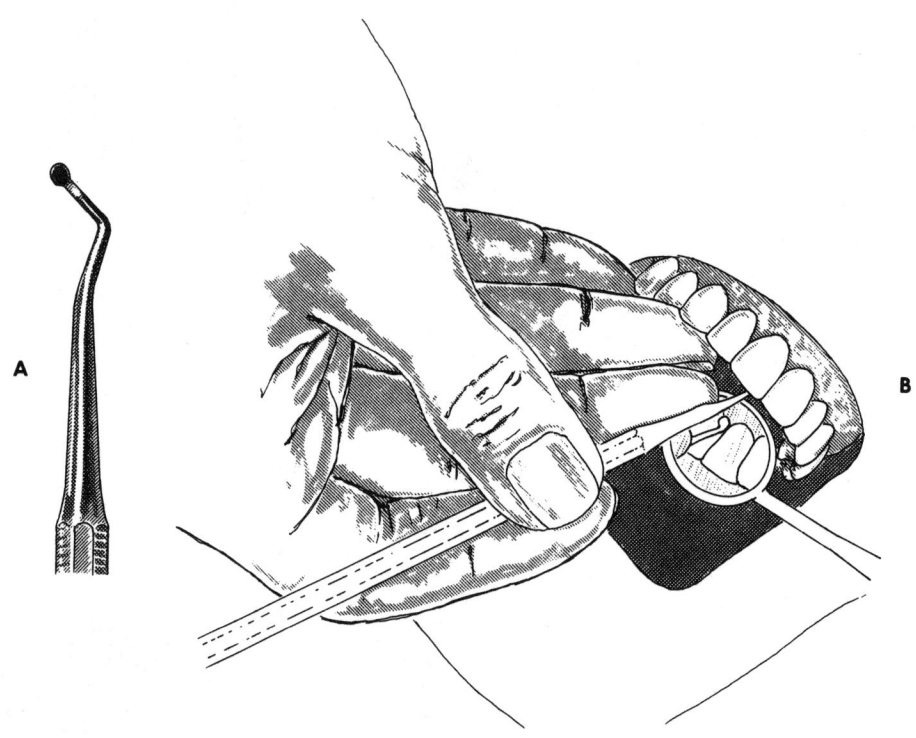

Fig. 4-14

5 ROTARY INSTRUMENTS

D. Joan Holzhauer
Peter Yaman

Rotary instruments perform the greatest percent of the work in dentistry. This includes five basic procedures: cutting, abrading, burnishing, finishing, and polishing. Before the evolution of rotary instruments, hand cutting instruments such as chisels and excavators were used for removal of enamel and dentin.

A steel shank with a cutting head on one end and a knob on the opposite end was used in 1846 as the first rotary cutting instrument. By placing the knob in the palm of the hand and rotating the shank with the thumb and forefinger, and the bur head revolved, thus removing tooth tissue.

Many drilling devices appeared over the next 20 years. Morrison's foot engine (1871) introduced a new concept in tooth cutting. The foot engine provided the first power-driven handpiece, which reached a speed greater than 700 rpm, inadequate by modern standards but a significant improvement over the existing technology.

The electric dental engine, the next stage of development, replaced the foot treadle and appeared about 1880. It reached a speed of 3000 to 4000 rpm, introducing the problem of frictional heat.

In the last 20 years revolutionary improvements have been made in the dental handpieces. With the introduction of the turbine handpiece, water coolant, and still higher speeds, the efficiency of all operative dental procedures has increased, and the discomforts of pain, heat, vibration, and cutting pressures have been greatly reduced or eliminated.

HANDPIECES
Low-speed handpieces

Physical characteristics
1. Rotational speed less than 10,000 rpm.
2. Manufactured as a straight handpiece or as a contra-angle handpiece with a friction-grip head or a latch head.

STRAIGHT HANDPIECE (Fig. 5-1)

Physical characteristics
1. Straight, tubular shape, but varies in length and diameter.
2. Driven by electricity or air.
3. Bur aligned in the same axis as the handpiece.

Use
1. Mainly for laboratory procedures.
2. Clinically for finishing and polishing procedures and for occlusal adjustments.

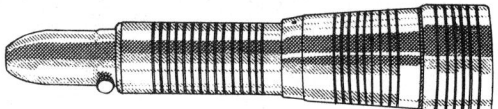

Fig. 5-1

ROTARY INSTRUMENTS

CONTRA-ANGLE HANDPIECE (Fig. 5-2, A)
Physical characteristics
1. Tubular-shaped mechanism, with a friction-grip head or latch head attachment.
2. Bur aligned at a right angle to the long axis of the handpiece.
3. Friction-grip head (Fig. 5-2, B) requires a special tool to place and remove the bur. Bur held in place by its frictional fit against a chuck inside the head.
4. Latch head (Fig. 5-2, C) has a latch mechanism to hold the bur. Latch is opened to allow the bur to seat into position. Latch is then closed around the bur to lock it into the head.

Use
1. To refine cavity preparation.
2. To remove caries.
3. For finishing and polishing.

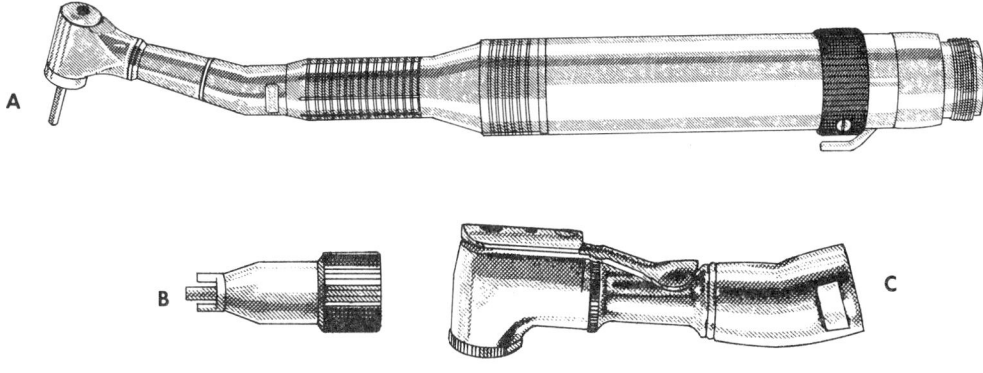

Fig. 5-2

High-speed handpiece
(Fig. 5-3)

Physical characteristics
1. Tubular shaped, with a slight angulation between the head and the shaft.
2. Available in varying diameters and lengths.
3. All air driven and capable of rotational speeds in excess of 350,000 rpm.
4. All with an air and water coolant.
5. Used only with friction-grip burs requiring a bur tool to place and remove the bur.
6. Bur aligned at a right angle to the head of the handpiece.

Use
For cavity preparation.

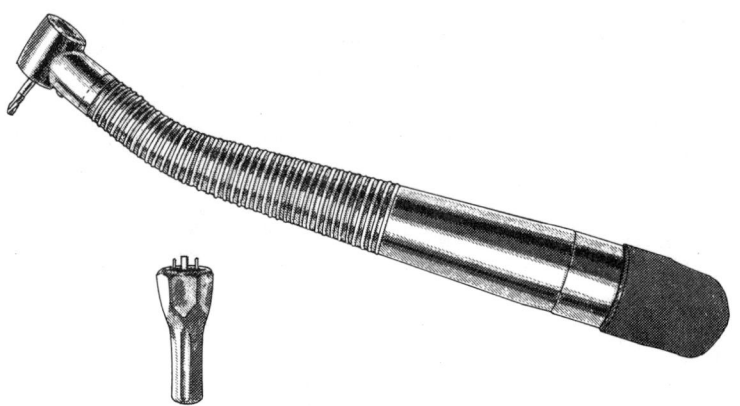

Fig. 5-3

ROTARY INSTRUMENTS

BURS   Rotary cutting instruments (burs) were made from carbon steel until 1947, when the tungsten carbide bur was introduced. The tungsten carbide bur proved to be twice as hard as the steel bur. The modern bur is a six-bladed cutting instrument produced from a blank by a special cutter. Burs are manufactured in hundreds of sizes, shapes, and types. The dental procedure being performed dictates the type of bur to be used. Each bur shape is identified by a numerical category. The burs within each category are numbered; the smaller the number, the smaller the size.

Each dental bur is made up of three parts (Fig. 5-4):
1. The shaft
2. The shank
3. The head

Three common instrument shaft designs are illustrated in Fig. 5-5: *A*, straight; *B*, latch; and *C*, friction-grip.

Table 1 shows basic bur shapes used in operative dentistry. These six basic types are manufactured in the three common shaft designs, although not in all the numerical sizes.

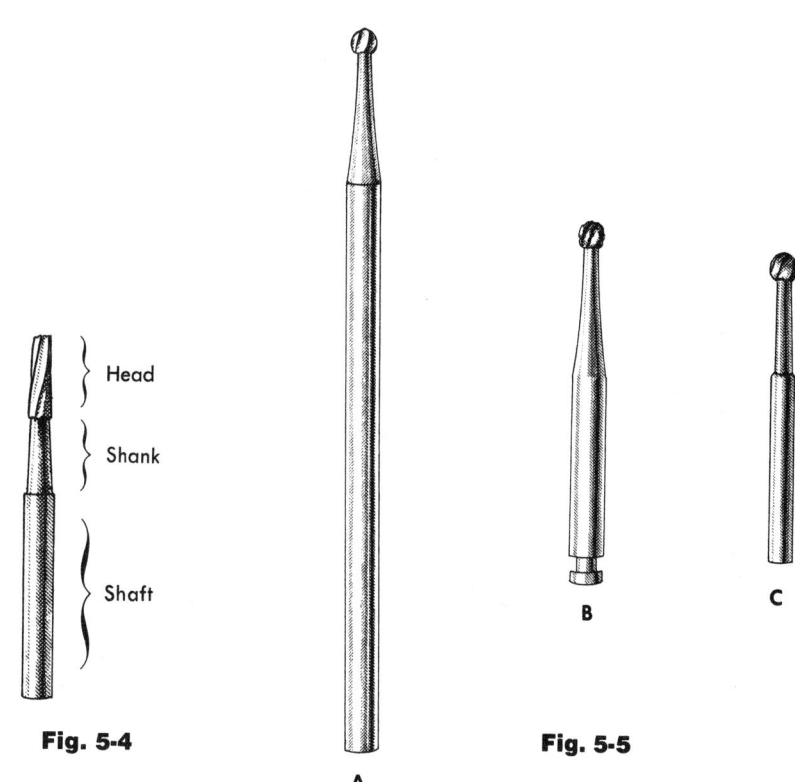

Fig. 5-4

Fig. 5-5

Table 1   **Basic bur shapes used in operative dentistry**

Type	Shape	Numerical category	Function
Inverted cone		33½, 34, 35, 37, 38, 39	Penetration: smaller burs (33½, 34) initiate penetration and outline cavity preparation
Round		¼, ½, 1, 2, 4, 6, 8	Penetration and excavation: smaller burs (¼, ½) for retentive grooves; medium burs (1, 2) for initial penetration and outline of cavity preparation; larger burs (4,6,8) for caries, removal
Plain fissure		55, 56, 57, 58	Extension and refinement of amalgam preparation
Tapered fissure		169, 170, 171	Extension and refinement of inlay and crown preparation
Crosscut Plain fissure		556, 557, 558	Low-speed bulk removal
Crosscut Tapered fissure		699, 700, 701	Low-speed bulk removal

ROTARY INSTRUMENTS

Plug finishing burs

Physical characteristics
1. Made of steel, with 10 blades instead of six.
2. The increased number of blades produces a smoother cutting action and leaves a smoother surface.
3. Fig. 5-6 illustrates various finishing burs: *A*, flame-shaped; *B*, 2-4-6 round; *C*, 2-4-6 pear-shaped; and *D*, wheel.

Use
1. At high speed for smoothing and beveling cast-gold cavity preparations.
2. Primarily to produce a smoother surface and to enhance the anatomy and marginal adaption of restorative materials during finishing procedures.

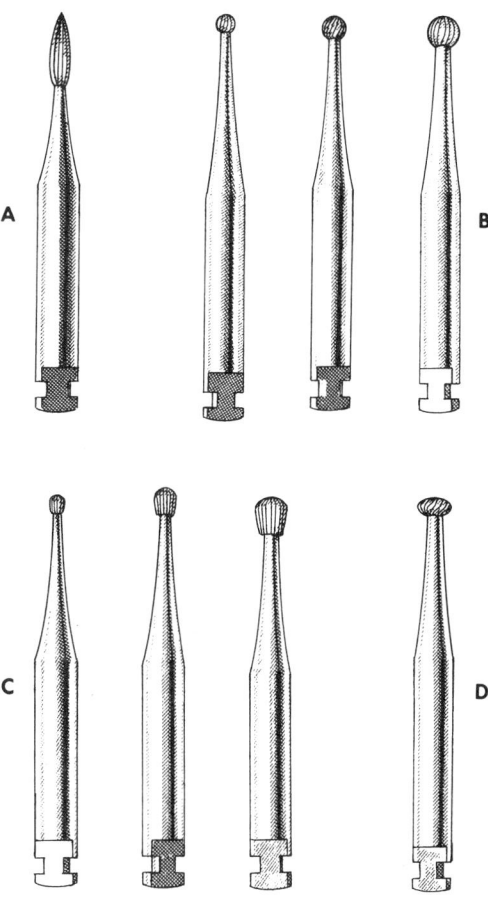

Fig. 5-6

OTHER ROTARY INSTRUMENTS
Diamond points (Fig. 5-7)

Physical characteristics
1. Abrasive cutting instrument with a metal blank and a metallic bonding material that holds the diamond powder onto the blank.
2. The grit varies from coarse to ultrafine (Fig. 5-7).
3. Available in a variety of sizes and shapes.

Use
1. Coarse grit for gross reduction of teeth during cavity preparation.
2. Fine grit for smoothing, finishing, and placement of bevels.

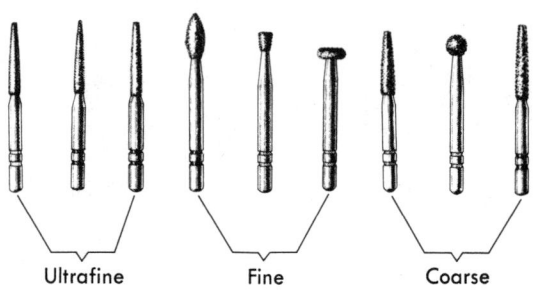

Fig. 5-7

Stones (Fig. 5-8) Mounted stones such as diamonds are included in the group of abrading and finishing rotary cutting instruments. The working end of the instrument is molded from a uniform mixture of abrasive and matrix. These instruments come in a full range of shapes and sizes.

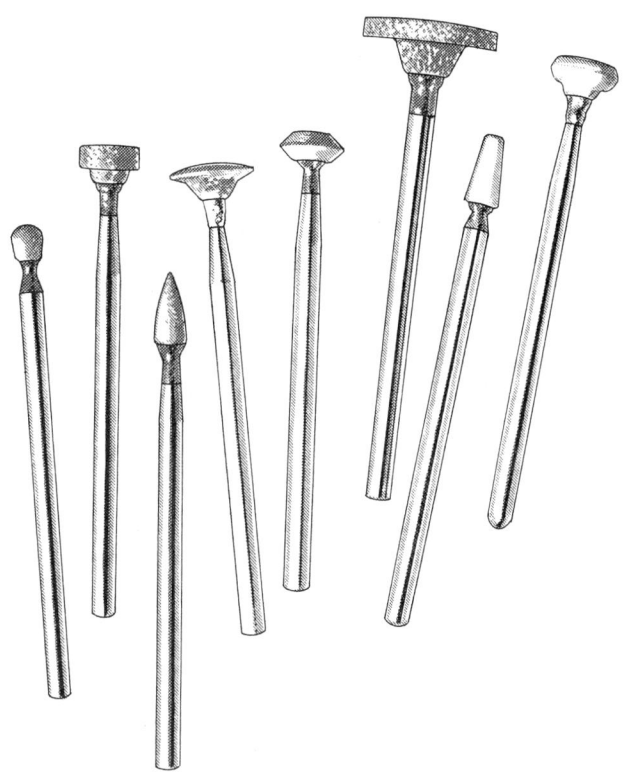

Fig. 5-8

GREEN STONES
Physical characteristics
1. Silicon carbide abrasive available in carefully controlled grits.
2. Produces a moderately rough surface.

Use
1. To initiate bulk removal of restorative material during finishing of amalgam and gold restorations.
2. For occlusal adjustments.

WHITE STONES
Physical characteristics
1. Dense aluminum oxide abrasive of fine texture.
2. Produces a smooth surface.

Use
To smooth restorative materials during final finishing.

Discs (Fig. 5-9)

Physical characteristics
1. Group of abrasive-coated instruments.
2. Flexible, molded, metal backed, or diamond coated.
3. Flat, concave, or convex (Fig. 5-10) and perforated or nonperforated.
4. Available in a large variety of grits; the abrasive coating can be either synthetic or natural, such as silicon carbide, sand, garnet, or quartz.
5. Size ranges from ¼ to ⅞ inch (0.6 to 2.3 cm).
6. Mounted either for a snap-on or a screw-on mandrel.

Use
1. Applied to the proximal surfaces and buccal and lingual contours of the teeth for refining cavity preparations and finishing and polishing restorations.
2. Soft backing of flexible discs should be flexed to allow the disc to contour to the tooth and restoration.

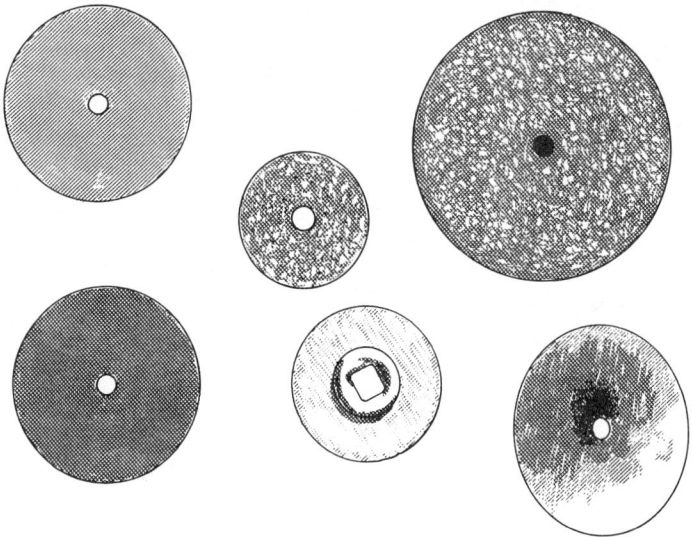

Fig. 5-9

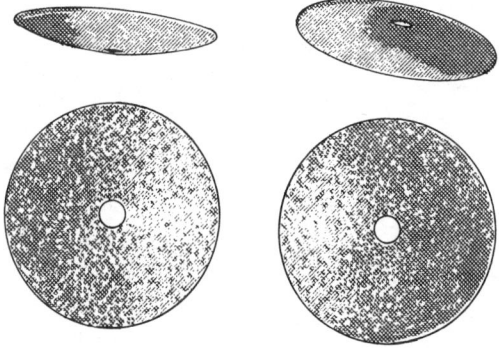

Fig. 5-10

ROTARY INSTRUMENTS

Wheels (Fig. 5-11)

Physical characteristics
1. Molded abrasive instruments.
2. Most common matrix materials are phenolic resins and rubber.
3. The rubber-bonded wheel allows for flexibility.
4. Silicone carbide and aluminous oxide are two types of abrasives bonded to a matrix.
5. Wheels come in various thicknesses, as well as in different diameters and grits.

Use
1. Primarily for laboratory procedures.
2. For finishing and polishing; extreme care must be exercised when used orally because a great deal of heat can be generated on the teeth.

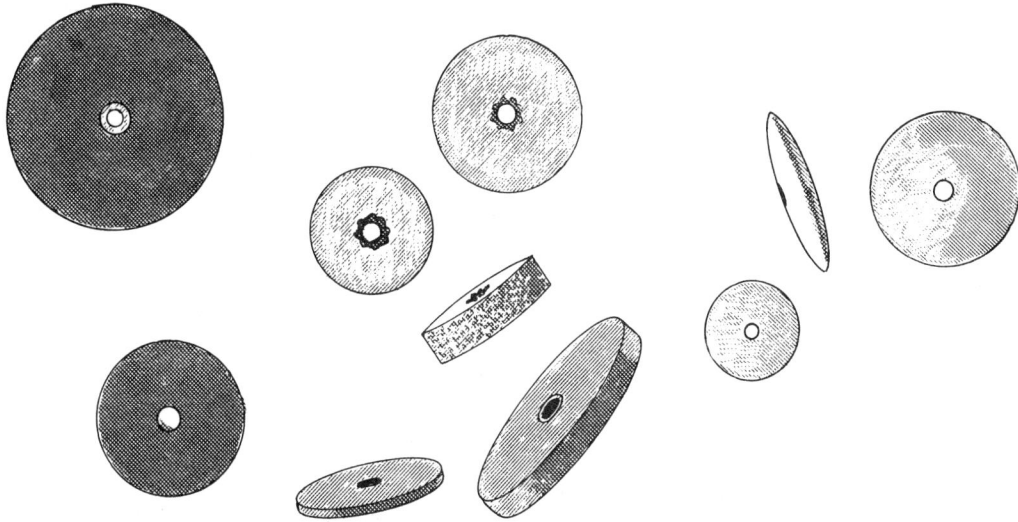

Fig. 5-11

Mandrels

Physical characteristics
1. Standard sizes for straight mandrels come with either a screw head or a snap head in the standard sizes of straight handpieces or latch-head handpieces.
2. Fig. 5-12 illustrates various mandrels: *A*, latch head, snap; *B*, straight handpiece, snap; *C*, latch head, screw; *D*, friction-grip head, screw; *E*, straight handpiece, screw; *F*, straight handpiece, pinhead screw; *G*, latch head, pinhead screw; and *H*, straight handpiece, extra-long, 3½-in (8.8-cm) screw.

Use
To hold discs and wheels in the handpiece.

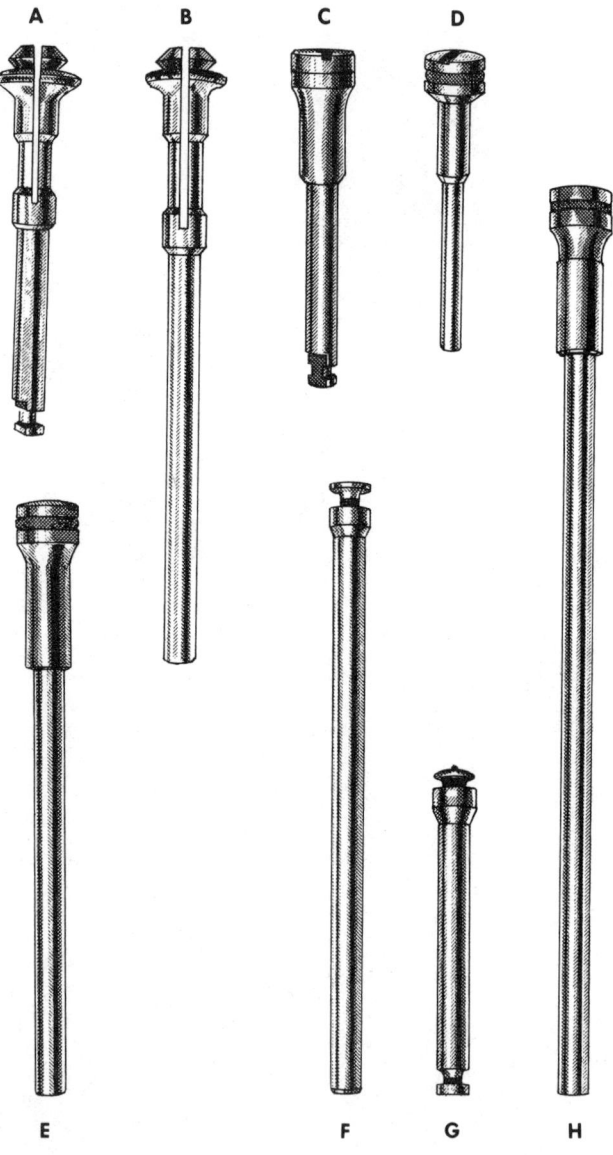

Fig. 5-12

6 AMALGAM CONDENSING AND COHESIVE GOLD INSTRUMENTS

Harvey Schield
Henry E. Brandau

There may be as many different brand-name amalgam condensers as there are manufacturers of hand and automatic dental instruments. Since the purpose of an amalgam condenser is to compress small increments of plastic amalgam into rather standard cavity preparations, the differences between the various manufactured instruments are usually quite minor. Such differences may involve the shape of the shaft, weight of the instrument, number of instruments in a set, angulation of the shank, and shape of the condensing surface.

Although the use of automatic condensing instruments has become popular for many operators, appropriate hand condensers are still just as effective and reliable. Emphasis must be placed on proper selection and efficiency. An oversight in these important areas will doom the amalgam regardless of the condensing method used.

AMALGAM CONDENSING INSTRUMENTS

A set of amalgam condensers offers a variety of shapes and sizes. Fig. 6-1 illustrates six different sets with slight variations in the shaft and condensing face. The face or nib (Fig. 6-2) of amalgam condensers is usually smooth, but there are condensers that have a serrated face thought to increase the surface area of the face and thus increase the condensing effectiveness. Neither type seems to significantly enhance the physical properties of an amalgam. The serrated face, however, often becomes clogged with residual amalgam and therefore presents a cleaning and maintenance problem, whereas a smooth face is easily maintained.

The shape of the nib or face of the most commonly used condensers varies between round and elliptic and from small to large. The edge of the nib may be rounded or angular, depending on the brand. This variance in nib contour is consistent with the internal shape of the cavity preparation, which is dependent on the shape of the rotary or hand instruments used to form the preparation. The preference of the operator regarding cavity design dictates the best-suited amalgam condenser.

There are other types of condensers, such as the Sweeney handle with interchangeable Miller points, that offer an even greater variety of shapes (Fig. 6-3). Round, ovoid, triangular, trapezoidal, or rectangular points that are also concave or angular from side to side provide the operator with the opportunity to maintain excellent condensation in many situations.

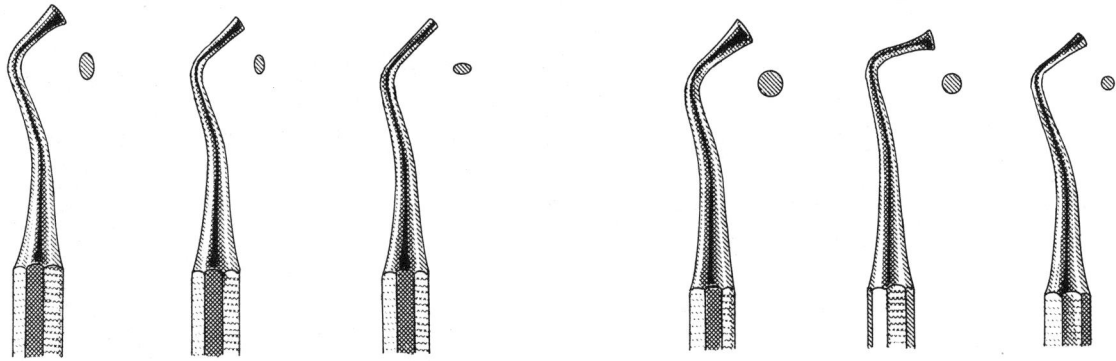

Fig. 6-1

AMALGAM CONDENSING AND COHESIVE GOLD INSTRUMENTS

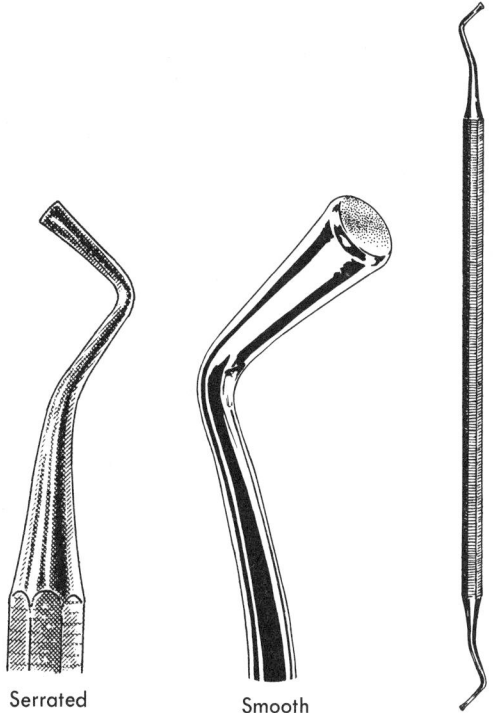

Serrated   Smooth

Fig. 6-2

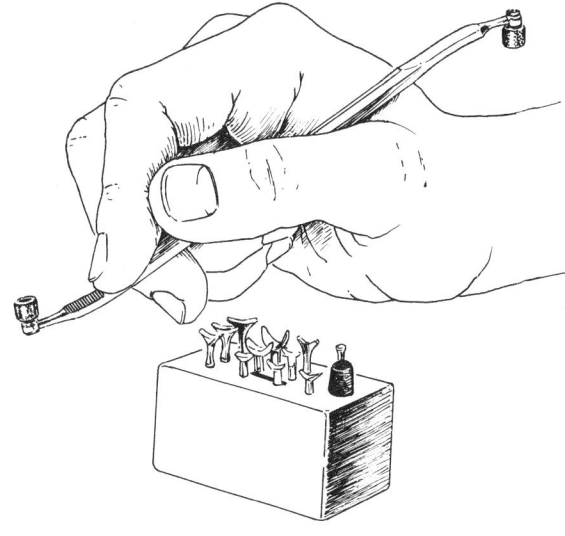

Fig. 6-3

Mechanical condensers

The automatic condensing devices, either vibratory or impact, may offer some advantages in speed of manipulation for certain operators, but they do not seem to improve the quality of the finished restoration. If an operator chooses an automatic device, extreme caution must be exercised to prevent teeth from chipping along a cavosurface margin during condensation procedures. Fig. 6-4 gives an example of a vibratory, automatic contra-angle and assorted condenser points. The point is latched into the contra-angle, and with eccentric forces delivered to the point, an up-and-down and lateral vibration results. The faster the engine is operated, the greater the magnitude of vibration. The points come in different sizes of round and triangular shapes, with a paddle-shaped point and a rounded, almost cone-shaped point available for less accessible areas. These latter two points are used more often in final contouring than in actual condensing.

As with any contra-angle, the automatic condenser contra-angle must be serviced routinely. Proper sterilization and care are essential to maintain consistent optimum operation. Although it is unusual for smooth-faced amalgam condensers to retain residual amalgam, careful examination is mandatory so that a restoration is not contaminated.

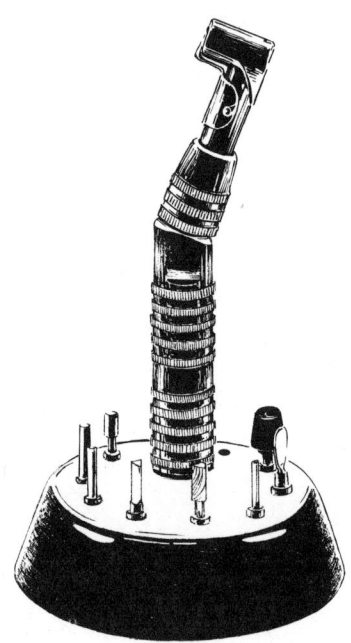

Fig. 6-4

AMALGAM CONDENSING AND COHESIVE GOLD INSTRUMENTS

Amalgam carrier (Fig. 6-5)

Physical characteristics
1. Single-ended instrument, or double-ended with large and small end.
2. Lever-action handle.

Use
To carry and dispense silver alloy materials into a cavity preparation.

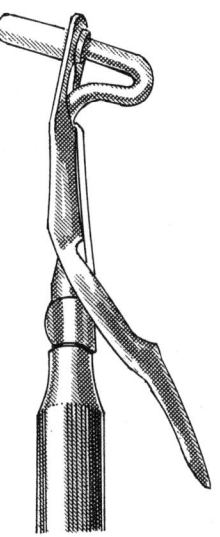

Fig. 6-5

Matrix retainers (Fig. 6-6)

Physical characteristics
1. A stainless steel instrument with two separate threading devices.
2. The matrix band inserted into the retainer and secured by tightening one of the threading devices.
3. After the matrix band is placed around the prepared tooth, the second threading device is turned to constrict and tighten the band.
4. *Tofflemire* retainers are illustrated in Fig. 6-6, with straight angle and contra-angle.
5. *Ivory* retainers are shown in Fig. 6-7: *A*, Ivory #9 and *B*, Ivory #1.

Use
To maintain stability of the matrix band during condensation of the silver alloy material.

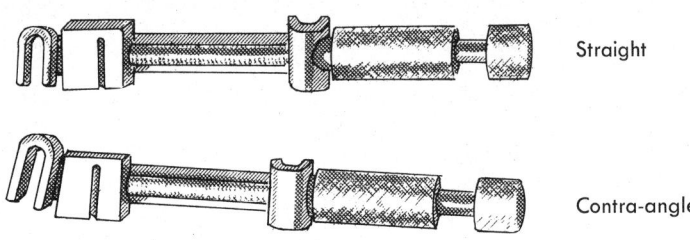

Straight

Contra-angle

Tofflemire retainers

Fig. 6-6

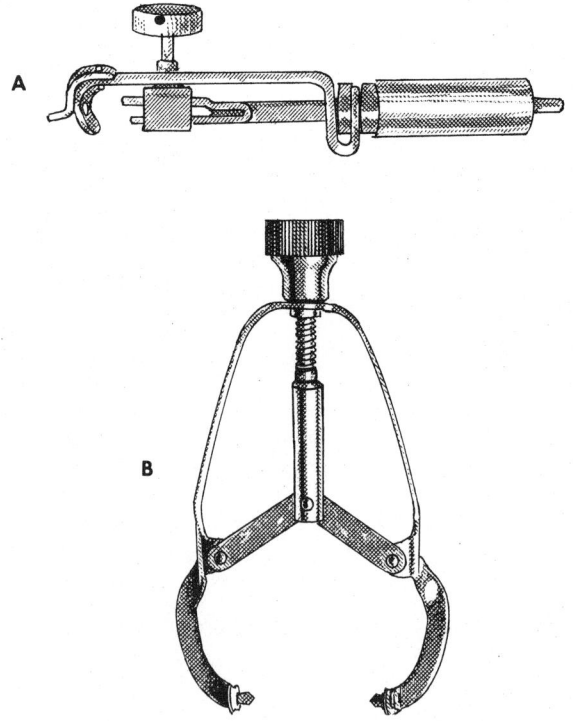

Fig. 6-7

AMALGAM CONDENSING AND COHESIVE GOLD INSTRUMENTS

Matrices (Fig. 6-8)

Physical characteristics
1. Manufactured in various thicknesses of stainless or carbon steel.
2. Range of thickness: .0015 to .0030 inch (.0375 to .0750 mm). The thinner matrices usually most desirable.

Use

Necessary for preparations of two or more surfaces involving a proximal surface.

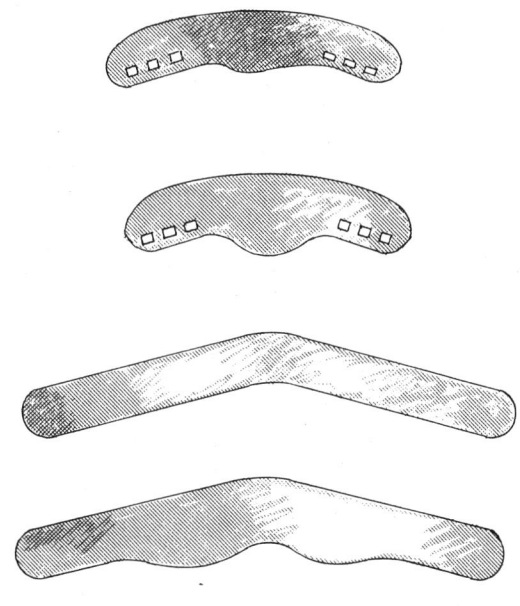

Fig. 6-8

COHESIVE GOLD INSTRUMENTS

The different forms of cohesive gold available for dental restorative purposes are fibrous foil, crystalline (mat), encapsulated powdered, and alloyed cohesive.

The manufacturer renders most cohesive golds semicohesive for ease in handling by treating the surface with a volatile ammonia gas. The use of heat to remove the protective ammonia gas makes the gold more cohesive.

Cleanliness of the instruments used in placing the cohesive gold restorations is important, since contamination may prevent coherence of the gold.

Alcohol lamp (Fig. 6-9)

Physical characteristics
1. Glass jar containing acetone-free alcohol.
2. Knob for adjusting cotton wick.
3. Protective cap for wick.

Use
For heating (annealing) the cohesive gold to eliminate moisture and gases and increase cohesiveness.

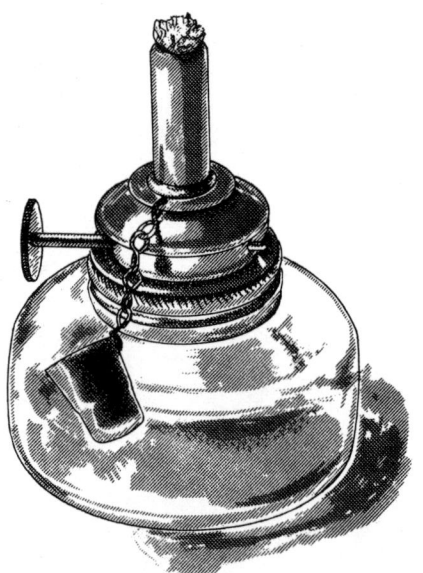

Fig. 6-9

AMALGAM CONDENSING AND COHESIVE GOLD INSTRUMENTS

Cohesive gold carrier
(Fig. 6-10)

Physical characteristics
Single-ended instrument, with working end needle-shaped or tined.

Use
To carry the pieces of cohesive gold from the bulk annealer or through the alcohol flame to the cavity preparation.

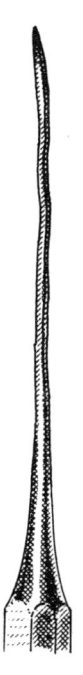

Fig. 6-10

Cohesive gold hand condenser (Fig. 6-11)

Physical characteristics
1. Available as a single-ended and long-handled or a double-ended instrument.
2. Straight or contra-angled shank.
3. Serrated working end available in various shapes and sizes.

Use
For condensation of cohesive gold through hand pressure or striking with a mallet.

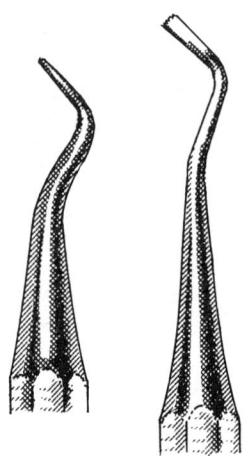

Fig. 6-11

AMALGAM CONDENSING AND COHESIVE GOLD INSTRUMENTS

Automatic hand condenser (Fig. 6-12, *A*) **and assorted condenser points** (Fig. 6-12, B)

Physical characteristics
1. The ends of the handle threaded to receive the various condenser points.
2. Mechanisms located on the handle for adjusting the length and force of the condensing blow.

Use

For condensation of cohesive gold through a push or pull motion that triggers the spring-loaded mechanism.

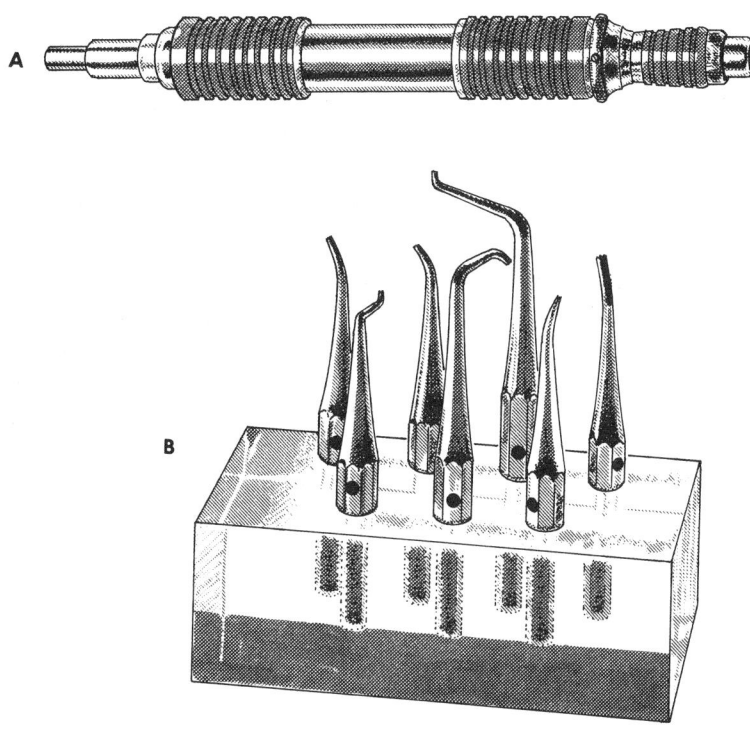

Fig. 6-12

Mechanical condenser
(Fig. 6-13)

Physical characteristics
1. Straight-angle or contra-angle handpiece available.
2. Controls adjust the frequency and the force of impact delivered to the condenser point.

Use
For condensation of cohesive gold through properly adjusted impact force and frequency and appropriate condenser points.

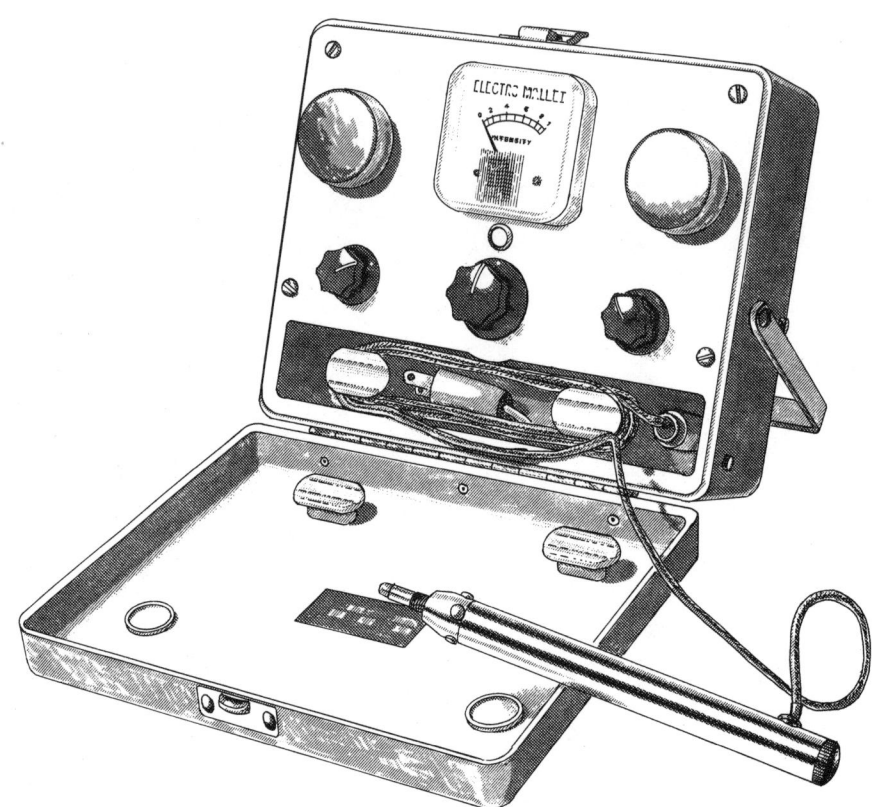

Fig. 6-13

AMALGAM CONDENSING AND COHESIVE GOLD INSTRUMENTS

Hand mallet (Fig. 6-14)

Physical characteristics
1. Hammer shaped.
2. Face either leather or nylon.

Use

To strike the handle of single-ended condensers with a series of light blows in condensation procedures.

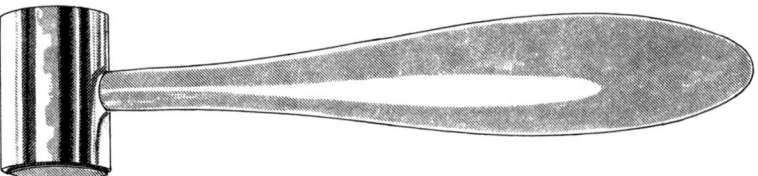

Fig. 6-14

Gold file (Fig. 6-15)

Physical characteristics
1. Single- or double-ended instrument.
2. Working end contains many small blades and is available in various shapes and sizes.

Use
To contour and finish cohesive gold restorations through a pull action that abrades the gold surface and develops the restoration contour.

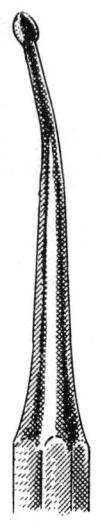

Fig. 6-15

AMALGAM CONDENSING AND COHESIVE GOLD INSTRUMENTS

Gold knife (Fig. 6-16)

Physical characteristics
1. Single-ended instrument.
2. Available in various shapes.
3. Working end has sharp, knifelike edge.

Use

To trim and contour the cohesive gold restoration through a controlled push or pull stroke.

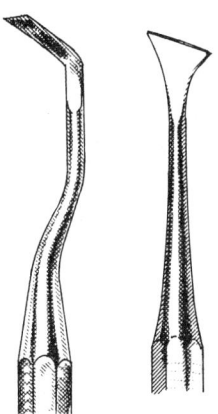

Fig. 6-16

Burnisher (Fig. 6-17)

Physical characteristics
1. Double-ended instrument.
2. Available in various shapes and sizes.
3. Smooth surface on working ends.

Use
To burnish the cohesive gold surface with a firm rubbing action.

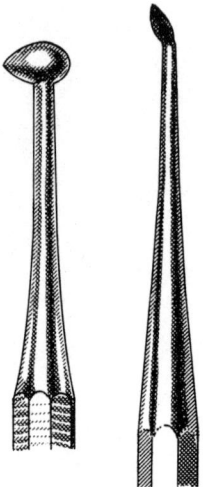

Fig. 6-17

AMALGAM CONDENSING AND COHESIVE GOLD INSTRUMENTS

Mechanical separator
(Fig. 6-18)

Physical characteristics
1. Single-bowed (Fig. 6-18, *A*) or doubled-bowed (Fig. 6-18, *B*) instrument.
2. Pointed jaws fit into the interproximal space.
3. With wrench for applying force to jaws (Fig. 6-18, *C*).

Use

To gain access to the interproximal surface by wedging the teeth apart with carefully applied pressure to the separator's jaws.

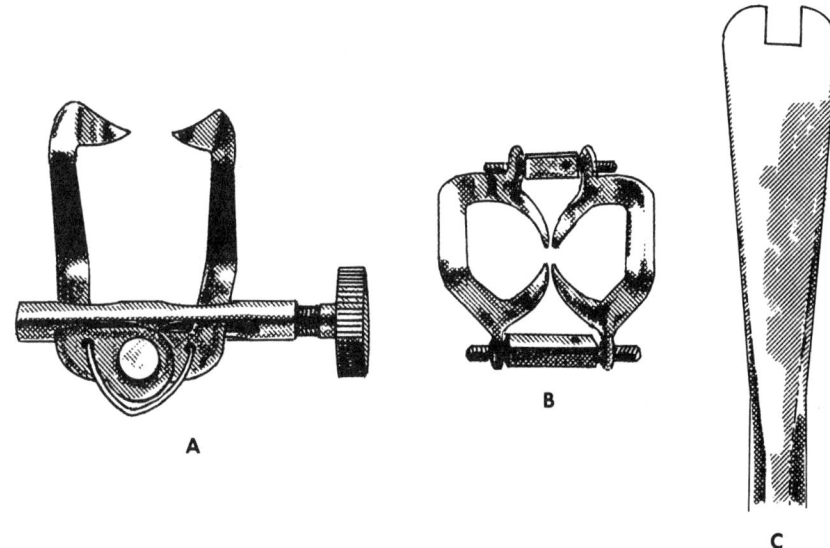

Fig. 6-18

7 ENDODONTIC INSTRUMENTS

John F. Corcoran

Endodontics involves the treatment of teeth with injured, diseased, or dead pulps. The purpose of endodontic treatment is to conserve these teeth so they can be restored and returned to function.

Conventional endodontic treatment is performed through an occlusal access opening in the tooth. Special instruments are necessary to debride the pulp canal, to prepare and shape the canal, and to place filling material.

Surgical endodontic treatment is usually done at the apex of the tooth because of the impracticality or impossibility of using conventional treatment. Special micro-sized instruments are needed to perform these procedures.

Long-shank spoon excavator (Fig. 7-1)

Physical characteristics
1. Similar to the spoon excavator used in restorative dentistry, except the shank is 10 mm in length compared to 5 mm on the conventional instrument.
2. Double-ended instrument.

Use
1. For curettage to the base of the pulp chamber.
2. For periapical curettage when access is limited or the roots are very small.

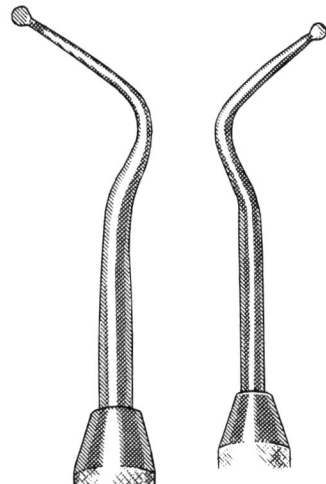

Fig. 7-1

Endodontic locking pliers
(Fig. 7-2)

Physical characteristics
Similar in design to conventional cotton forceps except:
1. Locking mechanism to keep forceps closed when finger pressure removed.
2. Grooved tip to hold root canal filling material or paper points.

Use
1. To facilitate the holding and placement of gutta-percha points and paper points into the root canal.
2. To grasp and transfer materials in and out of the oral cavity or the tooth.

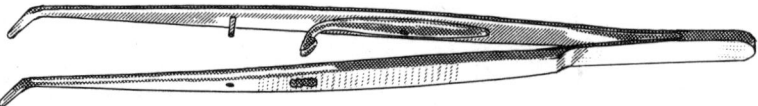

Fig. 7-2

ENDODONTIC INSTRUMENTS

Endodontic explorer
(Fig. 7-3)

Physical characteristics
1. Working ends straight and tapered, about 15 mm in length.
2. Double-ended instrument.

Use
To locate the small canal orifices in multicanaled teeth.

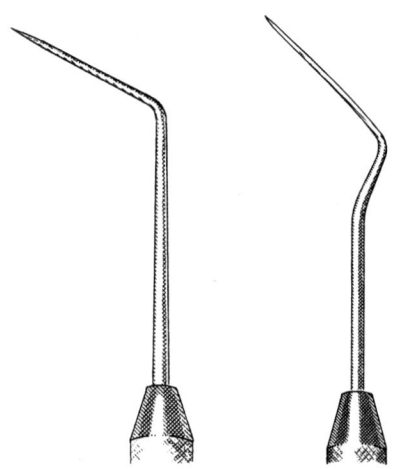

Fig. 7-3

Plastic instruments
(Fig. 7-4)

Physical characteristics
1. Double-ended instrument.
2. Paddle-shaped end (Fig. 7-4, A_1 and B_1) for carrying and placing.
3. Cylindrical end (Fig. 7-4, A_2 and B_2) for condensing or plugging.
4. Examples include MCE-1 (Fig. 7-4, A) and Woodson no. 2 (Fig. 7-4, B).

Use
1. To carry and place temporary filling materials.
2. To plug material into the root canal chamber.

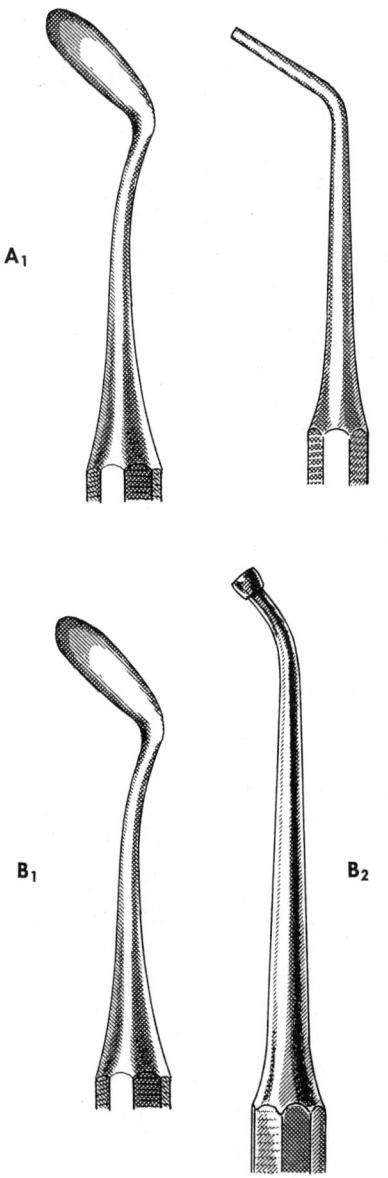

Fig. 7-4

ENDODONTIC INSTRUMENTS

Collar and crown scissors
(Fig. 7-5)

Physical characteristics
1. Scissors with small cutting blades.
2. Either curved or straight blades, with the curved preferred in endodontics.

Use

To cut paper points, silver cones, gutta-percha points, and so on. The curved blades allow the operator to cut the silver cones or gutta-percha closer to the occlusal reference on posterior teeth.

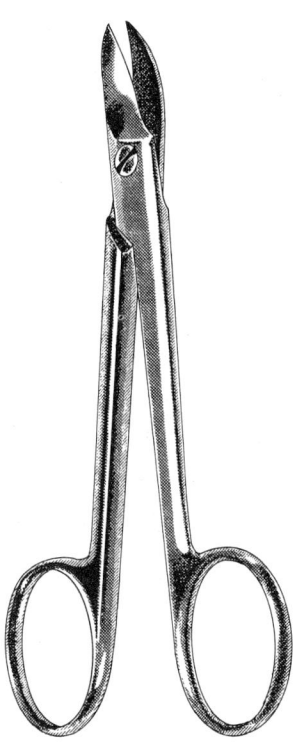

Fig. 7-5

Endodontic ruler
(Fig. 7-6, A)

Physical characteristics
1. Metal ruler with millimeter markings.
2. Attached to a metal ring that fits around the operator's finger for convenience.

Use
To measure the working length of the root canals; measurements taken from the portion of the first root canal file placed inside the tooth and transferred to subsequent instruments.

Application
Fig. 7-6, B.

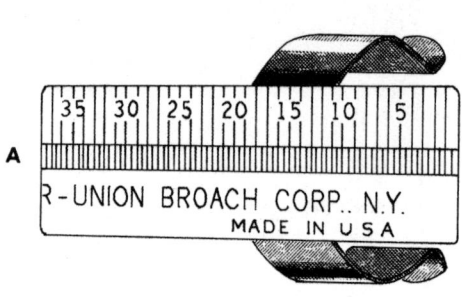
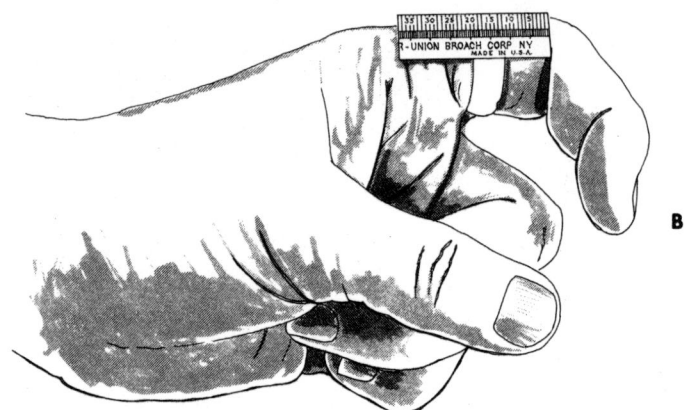

Fig. 7-6

ENDODONTIC INSTRUMENTS

Endodontic irrigating syringe (Fig. 7-7)

Physical characteristics
1. Usually a 2.5- to 5-ml (cc) plastic or glass Luer-Lok syringe.
2. Usually a 20- to 22-gauge needle bent about 45 degrees at the midpoint for easy access into the root canal.

Use

To carry irrigating materials into the root canal during the debriding phase of treatment.

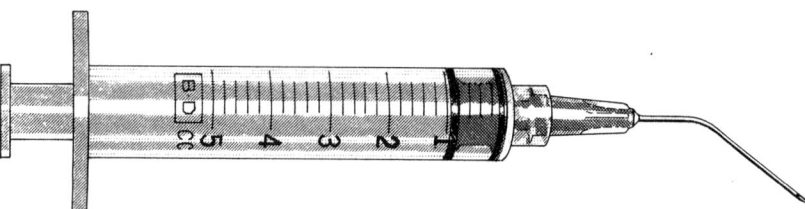

Fig. 7-7

Rubber dam frame
(Fig. 7-8)

Physical characteristics
1. A number available; the operator may have own preference.
2. Radiographic procedures much easier with plastic frames than metal ones.
3. Projections from the frames secure the rubber dam material in place.
4. Frames hold 5 × 5-inch (12.5 × 12.5-cm) rubber dam.
5. Three types: *A*, Young frame (metal); *B*, Starlite frame (plastic); and *C*, Nygard-Ostby frame (plastic).

Use
1. To isolate the tooth and root canal from contamination from the oral cavity.
2. To protect the oral cavity from irritating agents used in the root canal.
3. To protect the patient from aspirating an instrument or medicament that is accidently dropped.

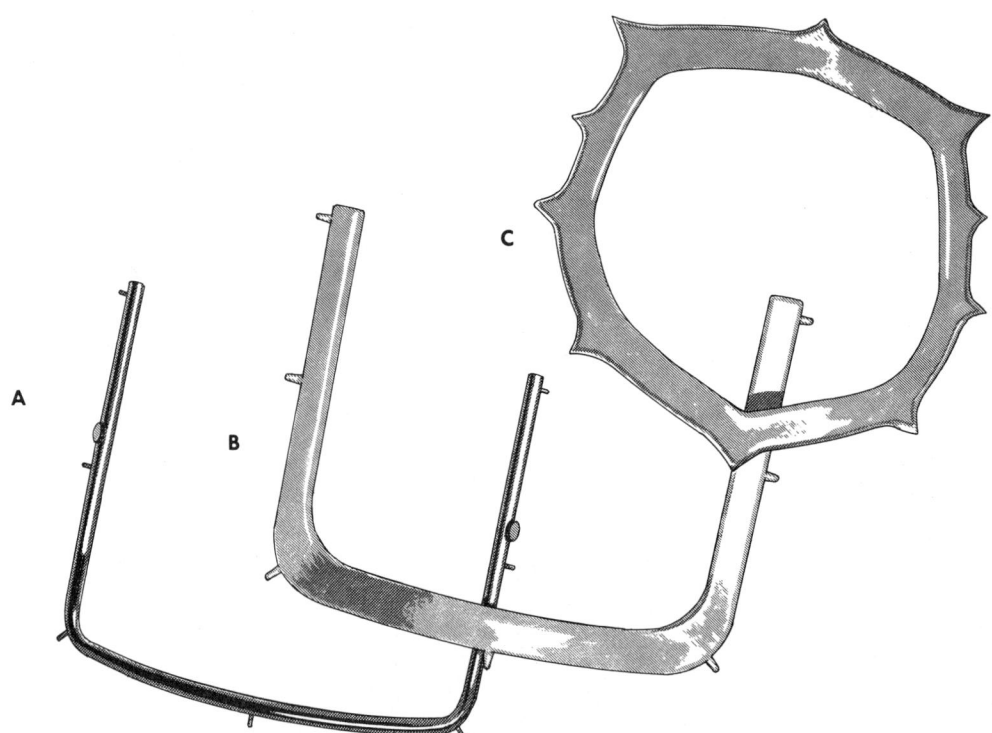

Fig. 7-8

ENDODONTIC INSTRUMENTS

Rubber dam clamps
(Fig. 7-9)

Physical characteristics
1. Clamps with wings preferable for endodontic procedures.
2. With the following clamps most teeth can be isolated for endodontic treatment: *A*, Ivory #9; *B*, Ivory #5; *C*, Ivory #14; and *D*, Ivory #1.

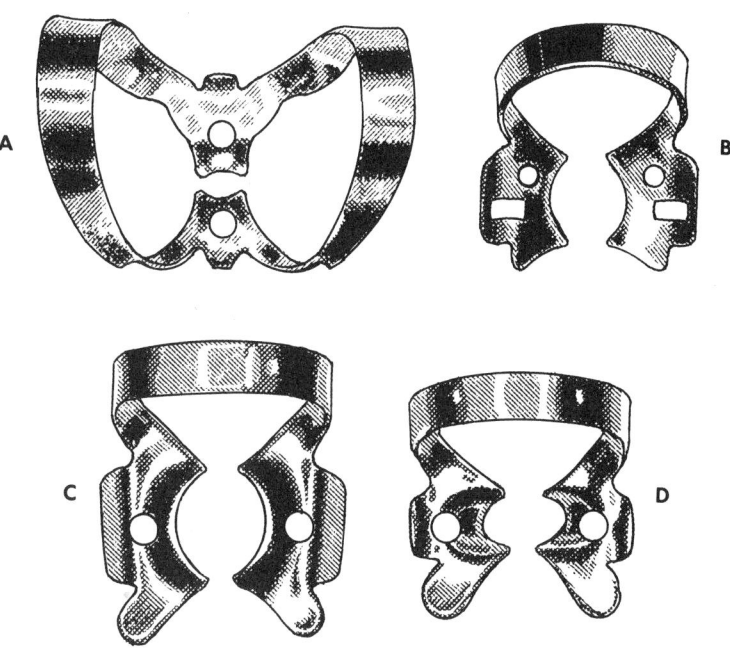

Fig. 7-9

Rubber dam forceps
(Fig. 7-10)

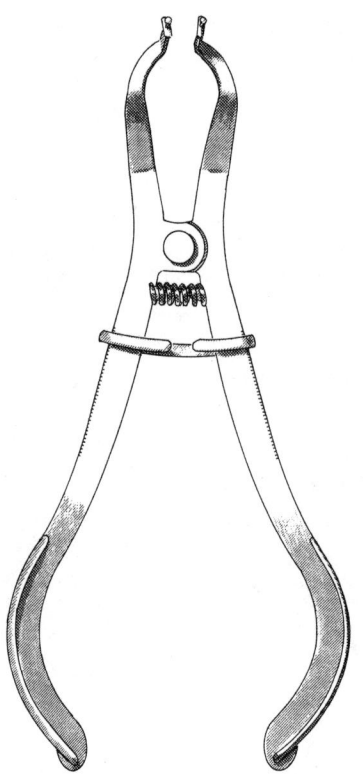

Fig. 7-10

Rubber dam punch
(Fig. 7-11)

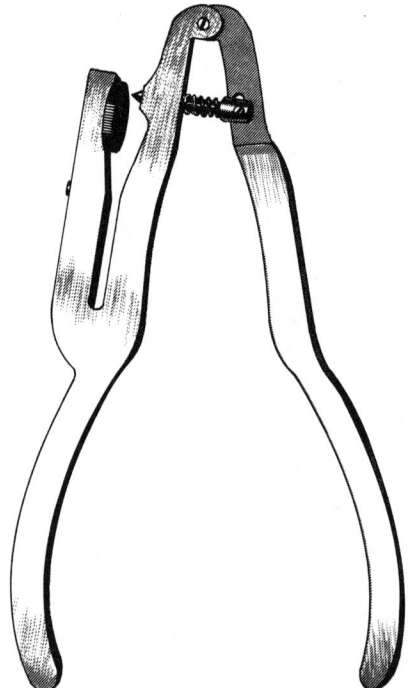

Fig. 7-11

ENDODONTIC INSTRUMENTS

Rubber dam Application
Fig. 7-12.

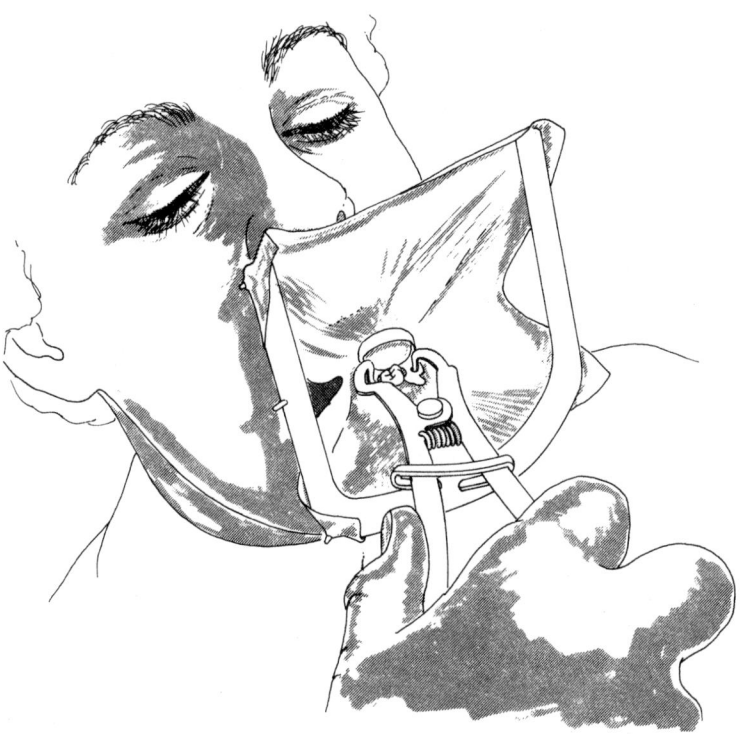

Fig. 7-12

Svedopter
(Fig. 7-13)

Use

To isolate a tooth impossible to clamp because of extensive caries or coronal fracture; used with cotton rolls (Chapter 3). The endodontic instruments threaded with dental floss in case they are accidentally dropped.

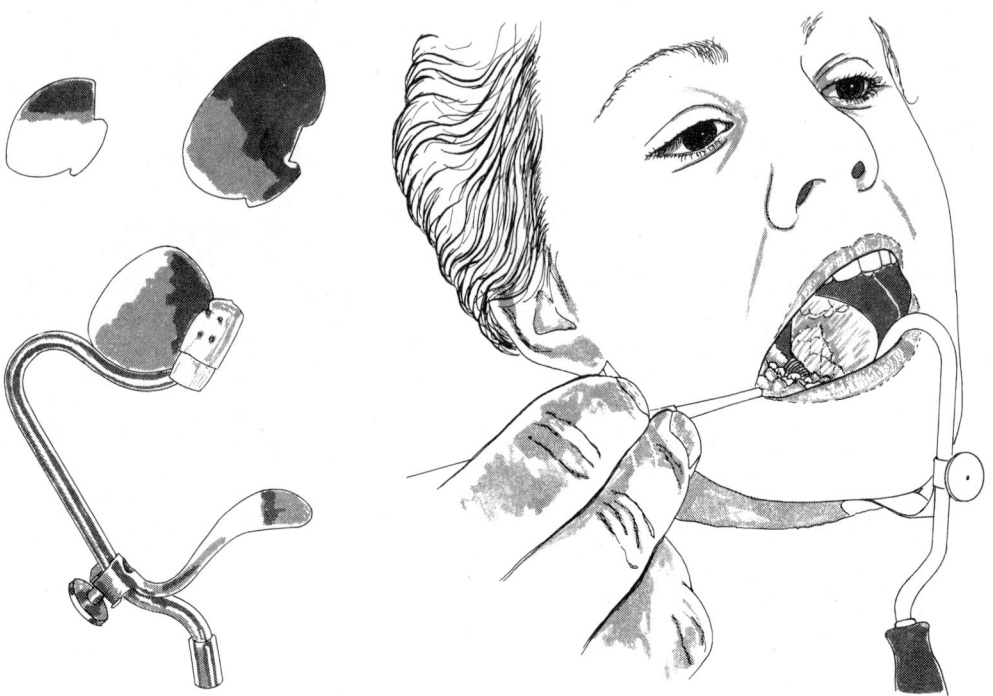

Fig. 7-13

ENDODONTIC INSTRUMENTS

Root canal files
(Fig. 7-14)

Physical characteristics

1. Instruments such as files used in the root canal available from most manufacturers in a standardized form (Table 2).
2. Handles color-coded according to the diameter to allow quick selection.
3. The diameter at D_2 is 0.30 mm larger than the diameter at D_1.
4. Designed with a uniform taper constant between D_1 and D_2.

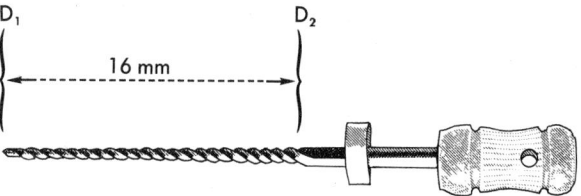

Fig. 7-14

Table 2 Standardized dental instrument data

Instrument number	Color	Diameter in mm at	
		D_1	D_2
8	Gray	0.08	0.38
10	Purple	0.10	0.40
15	White	0.15	0.45
20	Yellow	0.20	0.50
25	Red	0.25	0.55
30	Blue	0.30	0.60
35	Green	0.35	0.65
40	Black	0.40	0.70
45	White	0.45	0.75
50	Yellow	0.50	0.80
55	Red	0.55	0.85
60	Blue	0.60	0.90
70	Green	0.70	1.00
80	Black	0.80	1.10
90	White	0.90	1.20
100	Yellow	1.00	1.30
110	Red	1.10	1.40
120	Blue	1.20	1.50
130	Green	1.30	1.60
140	Black	1.40	1.70

INTRACANAL INSTRUMENTS

K-type file (Fig. 7-15)

Physical characteristics
1. Manufactured from a wire blank with a square diameter.
2. The blank is twisted, producing a series of cutting edges.

Use
1. To prepare the canal by placing the file in the canal, making a one-quarter turn clockwise, and withdrawing it.
2. Most common instrument for preparing the root canal.

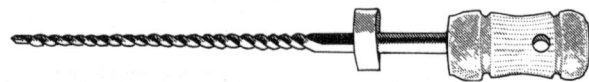

Fig. 7-15

Reamer (Fig. 7-16)

Physical characteristics
1. Manufactured from a wire blank with a triangular diameter.
2. When the blank is twisted, fewer cutting edges are produced.

Use
To cut the dentinal walls of the canal with a screwing movement.

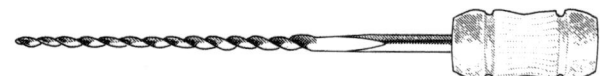

Fig. 7-16

Hedstrom files (Fig. 7-17)

Physical characteristics
1. Manufactured by a rotating cutter producing triangular segments in a round blank, creating an effective cutting instrument.
2. Major drawback is that it may fracture if it is rotated in the canal.

Use
To prepare the canal by placing the file into the canal and withdrawing it against the canal wall.

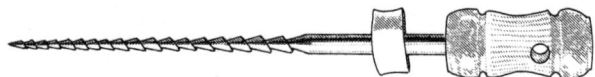

Fig. 7-17

ENDODONTIC INSTRUMENTS

Broach (Fig. 7-18)

Physical characteristics

Manufactured by notching the walls of a round blank.

Use

1. To engage and remove pulp tissue, cotton pellets, absorbent points, and other debris from the root canal.
2. Not used to prepare the canal because of the weakness of the manufactured barbs.

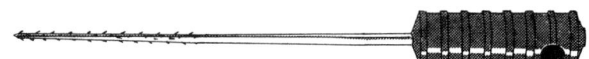

Fig. 7-18

Orifice opener (Fig. 7-19)

Use

To expand the size of the canal at its orifice once the canal is located. This permits easier placement of subsequent instruments and filling materials directly into the canal without bending them by hitting the tooth proper.

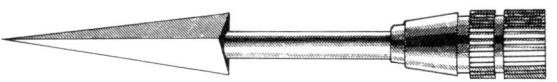

Fig. 7-19

ROTARY INSTRUMENTS

Gates Glidden drill (Fig. 7-20)

Use
1. Usually to expand the canal orifices for easier placement of instruments and filling materials directly into the canal proper.
2. Used by some practitioners to expand the coronal portion of the root canal during the biomechanical preparation phase in conjunction with hand-held files or reamers. If these instruments bind in the canal, they will readily fracture.

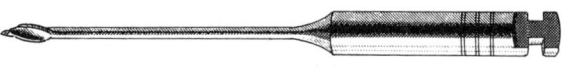

Fig. 7-20

Peeso reamer (Fig. 7-21)

Use
Primarily to open the diameter of the prepared root canal in the preparation of a post hole.

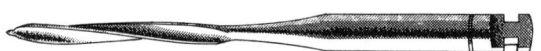

Fig. 7-21

Engine-driven reamer (Fig. 7-22)

Use
To prepare the root canal using a special handpiece designed for canal preparation.

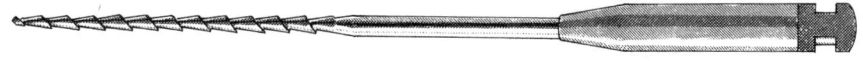

Fig. 7-22

CONTRA-ANGLES FOR CANAL PREPARATION

10:1 reduction contra-angle (Fig. 7-23)

Physical characteristics
Turns in a continuous circle.

Use
To prepare the canal using an engine reamer at a very slow speed.

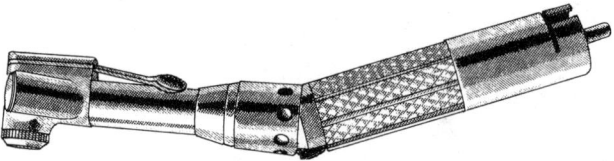

Fig. 7-23

ENDODONTIC INSTRUMENTS

Giromatic contra-angle (Fig. 7-24)

Physical characteristics

Operates with a reciprocating one-quarter turn movement.

Use

To prepare the canal using engine reamers.

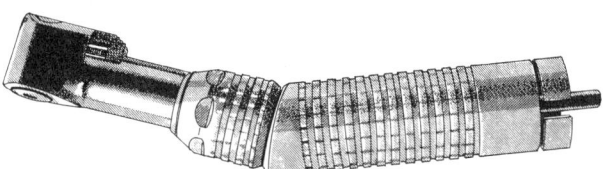

Fig. 7-24

Pfingst Racer contra-angle (Fig. 7-25, A)

Physical characteristics

Uses an up-and-down motion over a distance of 2.5 mm while oscillating with a one-quarter turn movement.

Use

To prepare the canals using 40-mm K-type files (Fig. 7-25, B).

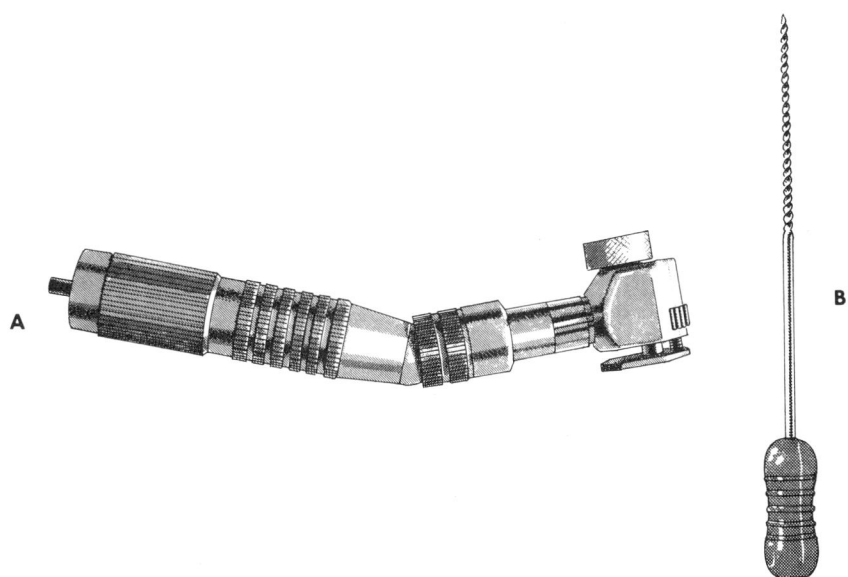

Fig. 7-25

ROOT CANAL OBTURATION INSTRUMENTS
Filling materials

1. *Silver cones* are produced as silver wires with the same taper as the root canal instruments (files and reamers) and are numbered in the same sizes as the instruments for canal preparation.
2. *Gutta-percha* is manufactured in two styles. Standardized gutta-percha cones are similar to the silver cones, with the uniform taper and diameter of the root canal instruments. Small A-type gutta-percha cones are used as auxiliary cones in the lateral condensation technique. Larger A-type gutta-percha cones are used in the vertical condensation technique.
3. *Paste fillings* are used to fill the root canal system in certain techniques.

Silver point pliers
(Fig. 7-26)

Physical characteristics
Straight or curved.

Use
1. To place silver cones into the root canals. Some operators prefer to use a straight or curved hemostat instead.
2. To remove the silver cones from the canals during retreatment provided the tip of the instrument is small enough.

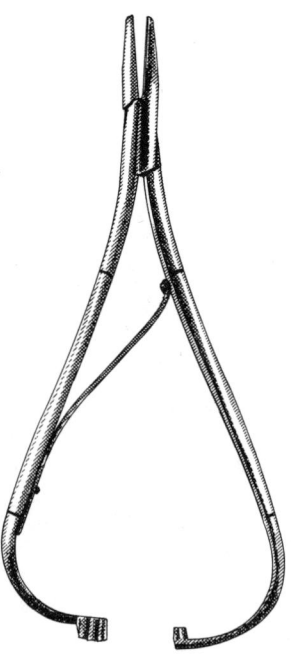

Fig. 7-26

ENDODONTIC INSTRUMENTS

D-11 (Fig. 7-27, A) **and no. 3** (Fig. 7-27, B) **endodontic spreaders**

Physical characteristics
1. Manufactured in various tip diameters and tapers.
2. Some of the tapers similar to the standardized gutta-percha points and others tapered similar to the A-type gutta-percha points.

Use

To assist in the lateral condensation technique of gutta-percha.

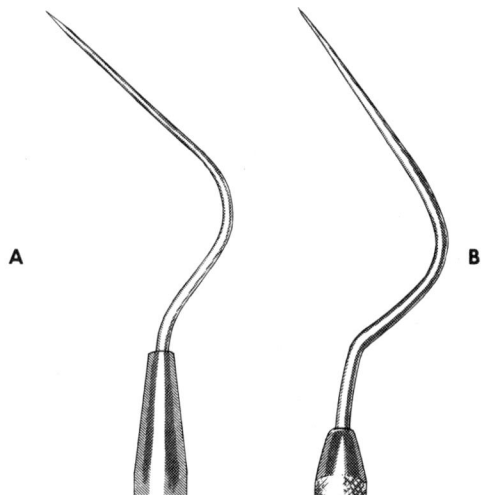

Fig. 7-27

Endodontic pluggers
(Fig. 7-28)

Physical characteristics
1. Manufactured in various tip diameters.
2. May have 5-mm segments scribed in the working end to identify its depth when inside the root canal.
3. Fig. 7-28 illustrates *A*, Luks pluggers and *B*, Shilder plugger.

Use
To assist in the techniques of vertical condensation of gutta-percha.

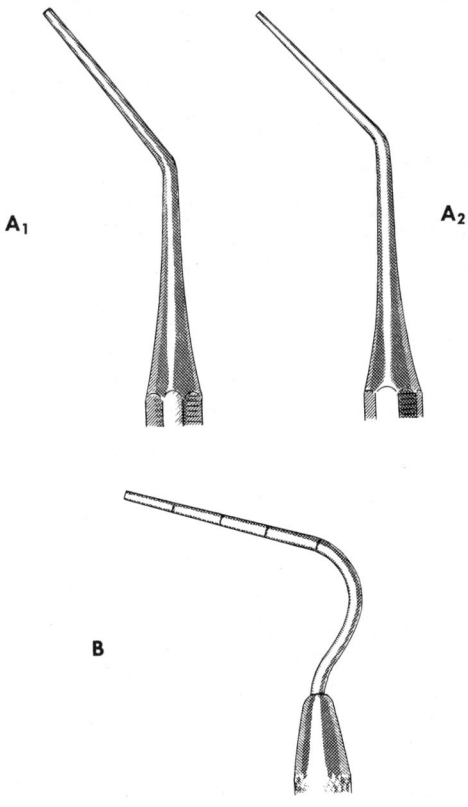

Fig. 7-28

ENDODONTIC INSTRUMENTS

Finger spreader (Fig. 7-29, A) **and finger plugger** (Fig. 7-29, B)

Physical characteristics
Manufactured in various tip diameters and tapers.

Use
To assist in root canal obturation in hard-to-reach areas of the mouth.

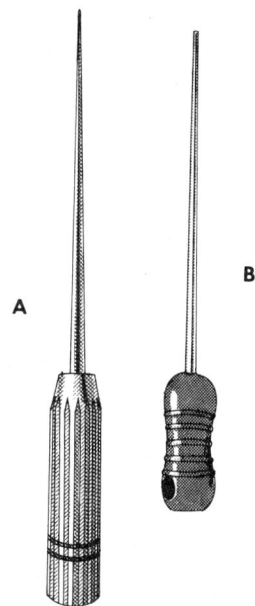

Fig. 7-29

Lentulo-type paste fillers
(Fig. 7-30)

Use
To place a paste filling into the root canal, by hand or by engine operation. Some operators prefer a K-type file or reamer.

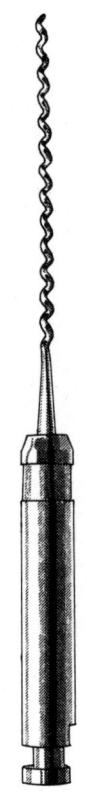

Fig. 7-30

ENDODONTIC INSTRUMENTS

ENDODONTIC PERIAPICAL SURGERY INSTRUMENTS

Surgical burs

Physical characteristics
Longer shaft (28 mm) than the normal friction-grip burs.

Use
1. To allow easier access and more visibility in the areas being treated.
2. A no. 6 round bur usually used for entering the cortical plate of bone.
3. A no. 558 cyclindrical crosscut fissure bur or a no. 701 tapered crosscut fissure bur used to remove the root end.
4. Smaller round burs used to make a preparation into the root end.

Retrograde filling instruments

The following micro-sized instruments are also designed to enable easier access during periapical surgery.

MICRO–CONTRA-ANGLE AND MICRO-SIZED BURS
Fig. 7-31.

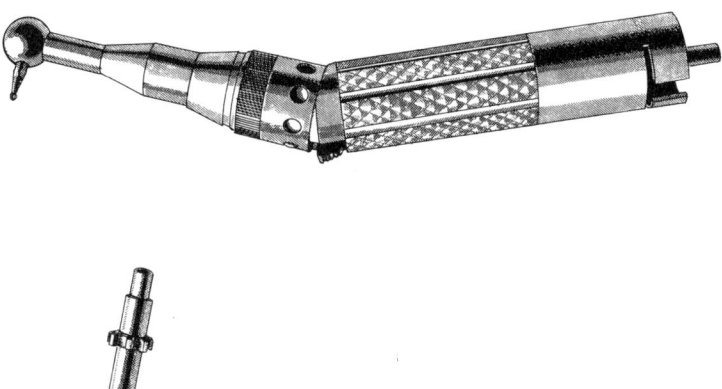

Fig. 7-31

MICRO-SIZED RETRO AMALGAM CARRIER
Fig. 7-32.

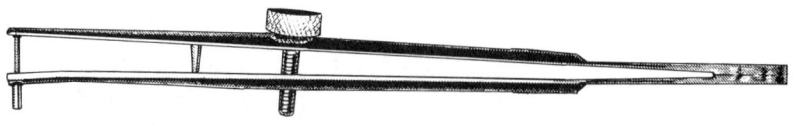

Fig. 7-32

MICRO-SIZED RETRO AMALGAM PLUGGERS
Fig. 7-33.

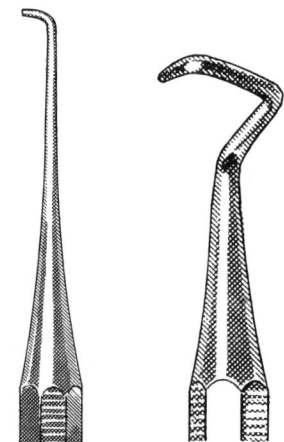

Fig. 7-33

8 ORTHODONTIC INSTRUMENTS

John B. Faust
Richard A. Johnson

Orthodontics is the part of dental practice that deals with the diagnosis and treatment of malocclusion and irregularities of the teeth and jaws. Procedures in orthodontics demand the use of many specially designed instruments, along with several borrowed from other areas in dentistry. The purpose of this chapter is to familiarize the dental team with the names, design, and function of these instruments.

Tweed arch-adjusting pliers (Fig. 8-1)

Physical characteristics
1. Opposing beaks parallel at 0.020-inch (0.50-mm) opening.
2. Beak surfaces available with smooth or scored tips.
3. Replaceable carbide insert tips for longer life.

Use
For holding and adjusting archwires, usually those with rectangular cross sections.

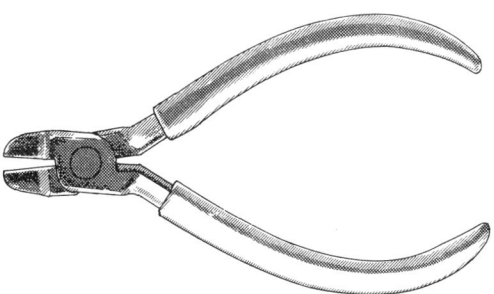

Fig. 8-1

Bird-beak (no. 139) pliers
(Fig. 8-2)

Physical characteristics
1. Conical and pyramidal opposing beaks, parallel at 0.020-inch (0.50-mm) opening.
2. Available with beaks of various length.

Use
For bending wire or seating separation springs.

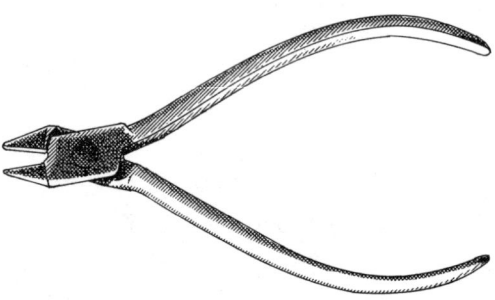

Fig. 8-2

ORTHODONTIC INSTRUMENTS

Nylon molar band seater (band biter) (Fig. 8-3, A)

Physical characteristics
1. Tips available in several shapes, serrated to provide positive grip on band edge.
2. Handle and tip one piece or with replaceable tip of nylon to cushion biting force.
3. Occasionally seen in metal-handled version.

Use
1. For seating and positioning bands.
2. For patient biting force.
3. Tip used to engage occlusal edge of band.

Mershon band pusher (Fig. 8-3, B)

Physical characteristics
1. Large, slightly tapering handle.
2. Long shank with the angulated tip.
3. The tip rectangular and serrated on all five sides to prevent slippage of the instrument during use.
4. Stainless steel construction.

Use
1. For positioning and seating the band properly on the tooth.
2. For burnishing or adapting the band edges around the tooth.
3. For tucking metal ligature "pigtails."

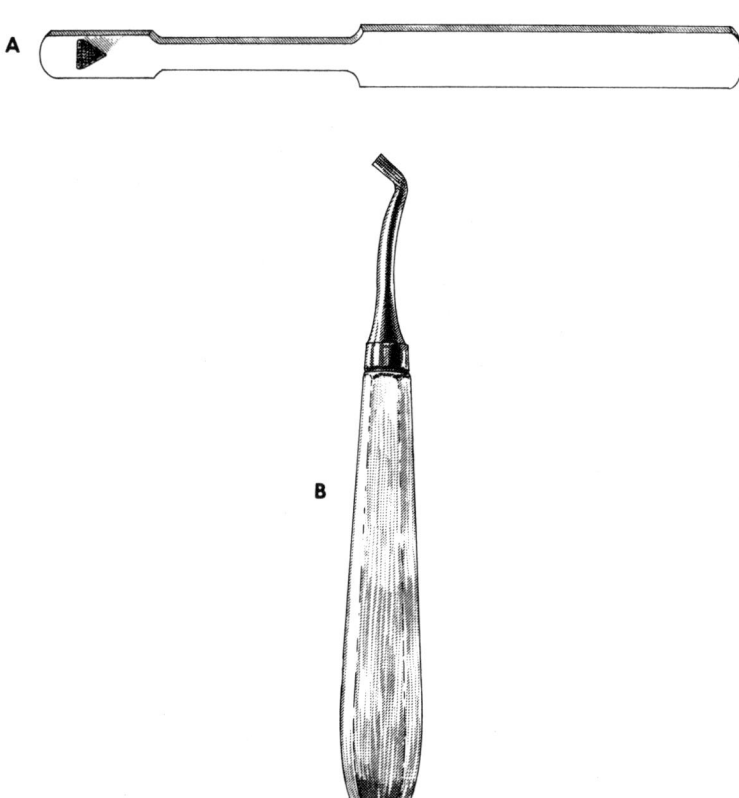

Fig. 8-3

Torquing key (Fig. 8-4)

Physical characteristics
1. Milled slot to hold wire and gripped handle to place or torque wire.
2. Double-ended with crosspiece and differently sized slots to accommodate various gauge wires.
3. Tips forked or of varying widths.

Use

For torquing archwires or placing wires completely into bracket slot.

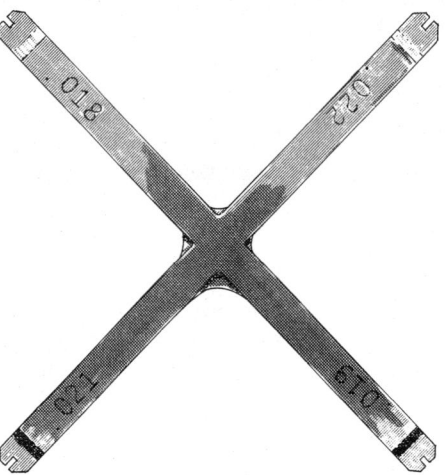

Fig. 8-4

ORTHODONTIC INSTRUMENTS

Serrated amalgam plugger (Fig. 8-5)

Physical characteristics
1. Angled, serrated tip for better control in pushing motion.
2. Available as single-ended instrument or double-ended in combination with ligature director or other tip by some orthodontic manufacturers.
3. Various lengths, angles, and diameter tips.

Use
1. To seat and position bands.
2. To tuck steel ligatures.

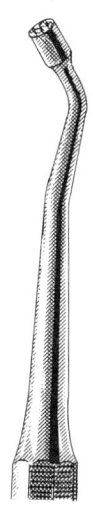

Fig. 8-5

Separating elastic pliers
(Fig. 8-6)

Physical characteristics
1. Reverse-action pliers with circular hinge.
2. Tapered, grooved, blunted tips to hold modules.
3. Angled beaks for better access.

Use
To stretch, hold, and place elastic separating modules by placing module over beaks.

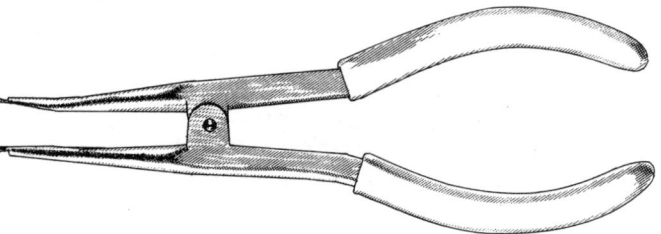

Fig. 8-6

ORTHODONTIC INSTRUMENTS

Triple-beaked pliers (Clasp adjusting) (Fig. 8-7)

Physical characteristics
1. Double-sectioned beak opposed by single beak, similar to face-bow–adjusting pliers.
2. Squeezing motion puts sharp bend in wire.
3. Box-jointed construction.

Use
For adjusting wires, particularly for offset bends in heavier wires such as on face-bows or retainers.

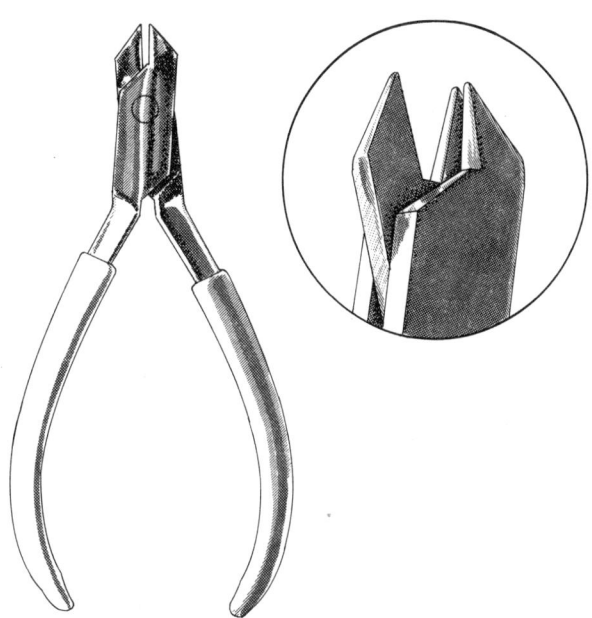

Fig. 8-7

Band burnisher ("B" burnisher)
(Fig. 8-8, A)

Physical characteristics
1. Heavy, hollow handle for palm grip, similar to Mershon band-adaptor.
2. Smooth or serrated tip.
3. Tip angled to shank and flattened for easier access to band margin under bracket wing.

Use
For burnishing and adapting margins of bands to the tooth at cementation.

Automatic band driver
(Fig. 8-8, B)

Physical characteristics
1. Single-ended instrument.
2. Large, hollow handle with spring that transmits a driving force to the tip when handle compressed and released.
3. Tips interchangeable, with either a straight, serrated tip or a curved tip.
4. Stainless steel construction.

Use
To aid in seating bands onto the teeth by delivering a pushing force with a spring-loaded tip.

Band-seating file

Physical characteristics
1. Chrome steel file with beveled tip.
2. Vinyl sleeve for tissue protection and operator grip.

Use
For seating, burnishing, or shaping band margins for better adaptation to tooth surfaces and grooves; used with a palm grip in a rotating, pushing motion.

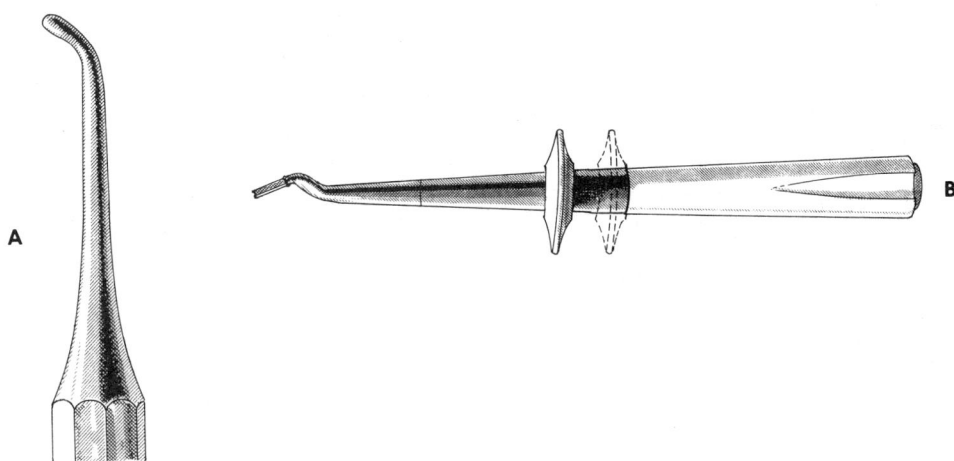

Fig. 8-8

Ligature director (Fig. 8-9)

Physical characteristics
1. Notched tips to hold wires.
2. Available in double-ended versions or in combination with other tips.
3. Tips straight or at angle for better access.

Use
1. To tuck and direct ligatures under archwire or bracket wings.
2. To push archwires or auxiliaries into position.

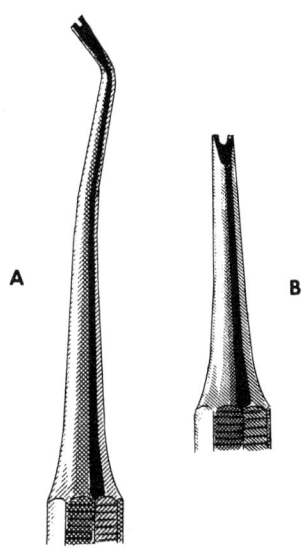

Fig. 8-9

Direct-bond brackets and bases (Fig. 8-10)

Physical characteristics
1. Laminated mesh surface on pads for adhesive grip; design of this mesh varies with the manufacturer.
2. Brackets welded to pad surface in position desired by the orthodontist.
3. Milled slots on brackets to hold archwires; size and shape of these slots vary with the orthodontic technique practiced.

Use
To provide a positive grip on the tooth for archwire or auxiliary attachment; attaches directly to the enamel surface with direct-bond adhesive cements.

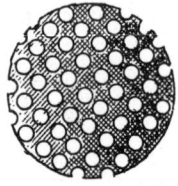
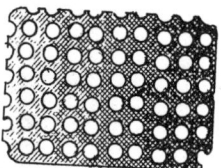
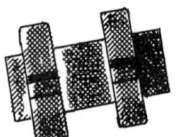

Fig. 8-10

Band-slitting and -removing pliers

Physical characteristics
1. Double-sided pliers.
2. Opposed horned beaks on crimping side.
3. Carbide cutting tips on slitting side.

Use
To remove cemented bands; horned end of pliers crimps the band occlusally and gingivally, allowing cutting edge to slit the band at the crimp.

Angulated bracket-removing pliers

Physical characteristics
1. Two opposing beaks angulated at 60 degrees from the handle.
2. Mirror-image jaws, with the cutting tips formed around a cylindrical opening.
3. Either wide or narrow jaws.

Use
For removing direct-bonded brackets from teeth by using peel and sheer forces at the bracket-cement junction.

ORTHODONTIC INSTRUMENTS

Howe utility pliers
(Fig. 8-11)

Physical characteristics

1. Two long, round beaks tapered to a pyramid shape and bowed to meet at the end by serrated pads.
2. The serrated pads at right angles to the long axis of the beaks; their diameter varies with the manufacturer.
3. Modified with a 45-degree offset angle toward the end of the beaks (E.T.M. offset utility pliers).
4. May have an adjustable screw joint.

Use

1. Mainly for gripping the archwires during placement and removal or making adjustment bends in the wire.
2. For seating bands, usually anterior ones.
3. For tying ligature wires.

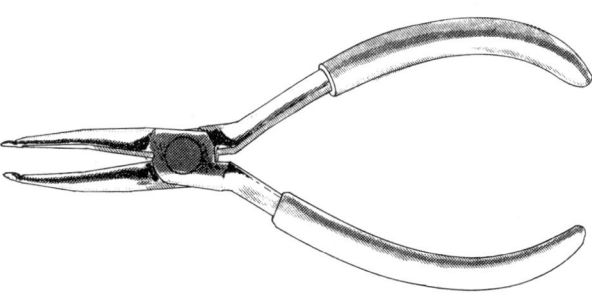

Fig. 8-11

Coon ligature-tying pliers
(Fig. 8-12)

Physical characteristics
1. Reverse-action pliers.
2. Opposing handles, shank, and tip (all one piece) joined just below the shank in a round, metal cylinder with a channel.
3. Opposing handles attached by a spring that holds them apart, causing the tips to touch when the pliers is passive.
4. Opposing tips forked for passage of the ligature wire and blunted.
5. As the handles are compressed, spreading the tips, the channel locks the end of the ligature wire automatically.
6. Stainless steel construction.

Use
For tying metal ligatures. Because of the reverse action, the initial twist and pressure are exerted at the bracket-archwire junction and then twisted away from bracket. This gives the ligature a tighter fit around the bracket, forcing the archwire completely into the slot.

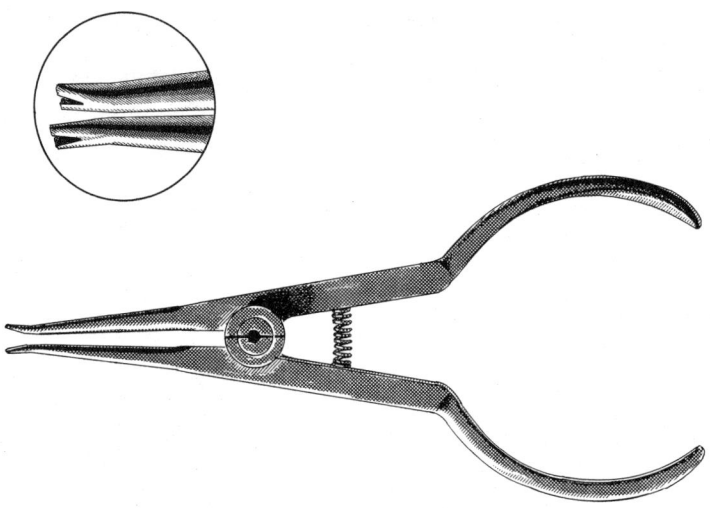

Fig. 8-12

ORTHODONTIC INSTRUMENTS

Posterior band-removing pliers (Fig. 8-13)

Physical characteristics
1. Two beaks, with a cylindrical, perpendicular nylon-tipped beak opposing a curved, flat-sided one.
2. Nylon tip replaceable.
3. Stainless steel beaks, with a carbide insert on the flat-sided gingival beak.

Use
To remove posterior bands from teeth during trial fitting or debanding. Nylon-tipped beak positioned on the occlusal surface, opposing beak positioned on the gingival portion of the band.

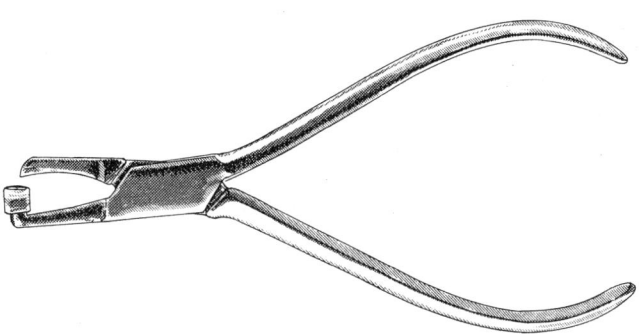

Fig. 8-13

Band-contouring pliers
(Fig. 8-14)

Physical characteristics
1. Two long, tapering, and slightly bowed beaks, with the opposing ends fitting together in a ball-and-socket manner.
2. Convex tip fits into opposing concave tip.
3. The diameter and shape of the tips vary with the manufacturer.
4. Stainless steel construction.

Use
For recontouring the orthodontic band for a better band adaptation around the tooth, as in amalgam matrix contouring.

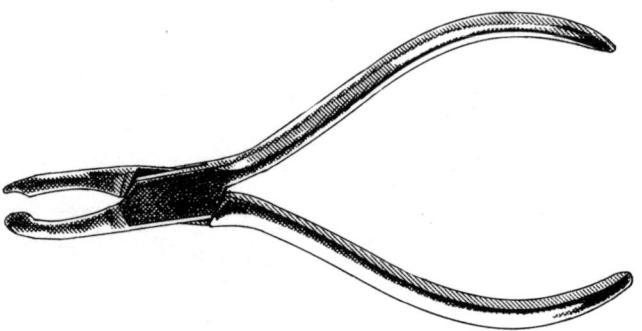

Fig. 8-14

Arch marker (pencil)

Physical characteristics
1. Wax pencil.
2. Variety of colors, with red or white the most common.
3. For use on either wet or dry surfaces.
4. Shows up well on stainless steel wire.

Use
For marking archwires to indicate location of adjustment loops or bends. Small files also occasionally used to mark archwires.

ORTHODONTIC INSTRUMENTS

Bands (Fig. 8-15)

Physical characteristics
1. Made of stainless steel.
2. Preformed and anatomically shaped to fit the teeth.
3. Fabricated in four major shapes for molars, bicuspids, cuspids, and incisors.
4. Each major shape comes in various sizes to accommodate individual tooth size variation.
5. Either plain or with buccal (brackets) or lingual (such as lingual buttons, sheaths, cleats, or seating lugs) attachments welded or soldered on the band.
6. Most bands have an occlusal-gingival taper to fit the tooth, with the incisal edge straight and the cervical edge contoured, similar to the cemento-enamel junction.
7. The band material varies from ductile and easy to deform to hard and less malleable.

Use

To serve as a means of holding or gripping to the tooth so that a bracket can be attached to it.

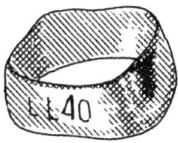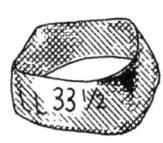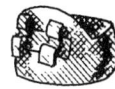

Fig. 8-15

Anterior-band-removing pliers (Fig. 8-16)

Physical characteristics
1. Two beaks, with the longer, flat-sided, curved beak used on the incisal edge of teeth opposing a shorter beak positioned on the gingival aspect of the band or bracket.
2. May have a nylon or rubber tip on the incisal beak to protect the incisal edge of the tooth from fracturing.
3. The beaks generally do not make contact when the handles are fully closed.
4. Stainless steel construction.

Use
To remove anterior bands from teeth.

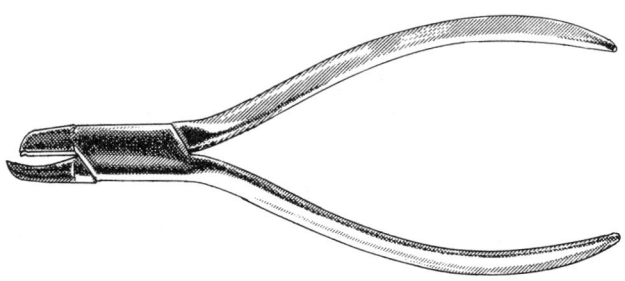

Fig. 8-16

ORTHODONTIC INSTRUMENTS

Orthodontic impression trays (Fig. 8-17, *A*)

Physical characteristics

1. Two main parts: the handle and the body. The handle either welded or riveted to the body.
2. Two types of bodies: (1) the maxillary body, which allows for coverage of the maxillary alveolar process and the palate; and (2) the mandibular body, which allows for coverage of the mandibular alveolar process.
3. Tray bodies either perforated, to allow better retention of the impression material to the tray, or nonperforated.
4. Available in different sizes to accommodate variable arch sizes.
5. The sides of the tray either extended to allow deeper impressions to the depth of the mucobuccal fold (good for study models) or maintained at regular height when only impressions of teeth needed and not full duplication of the alveolar process.
6. Most trays made from aluminum and flexible; others rigid. Some also Teflon coated for ease in cleaning.

Use

For taking impressions for either orthodontic study models (for diagnosis and treatment planning) or work models (for fabricating orthodontic appliances) (Fig. 8-17, *B*).

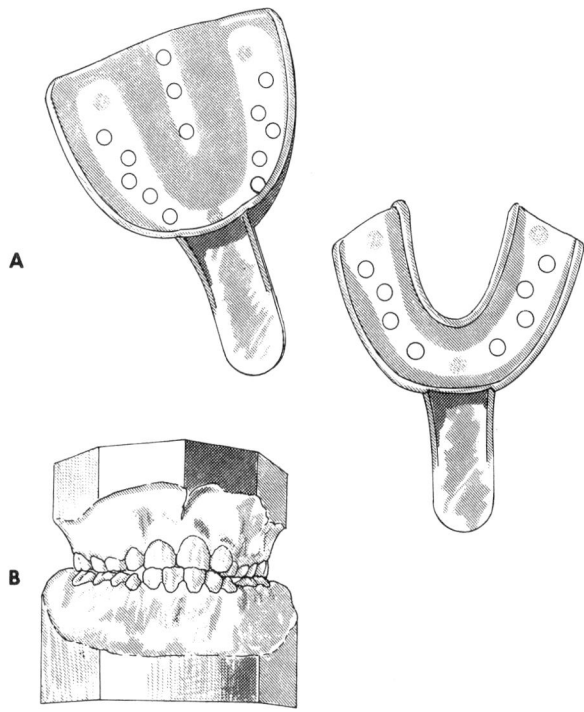

Fig. 8-17

Ligature-wire cutter
(Fig. 8-18)

Physical characteristics
1. Two tapered and pointed opposing beaks with sharp cutting edges.
2. The cutting edges may have carbide inserts that can be sharpened or replaced when dull or damaged without replacing the whole pliers.
3. Various cutting angles; straight or 15 degrees most common.
4. Taper and size of the tips vary with the manufacturer.
5. May have an adjustable screw joint.

Use
To cut soft ligature wires, generally up to 0.015 inch (0.375 mm) in diameter, and pins used to hold the archwires in the brackets.

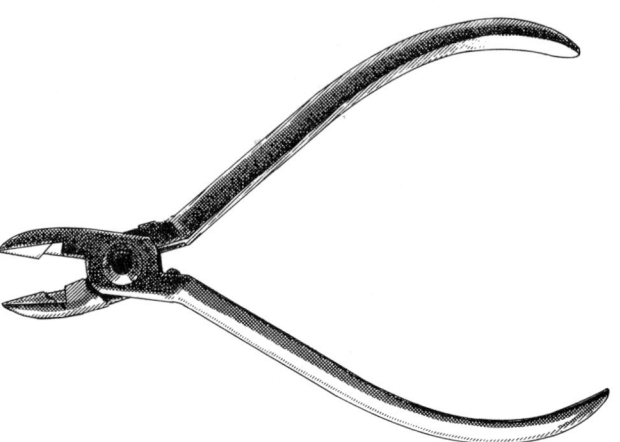

Fig. 8-18

Face-bow–adjusting pliers (Fig. 8-19)

Physical characteristics
1. Heavy-duty pliers.
2. Three parallel beaks: two opposing the one between them when the pliers is closed.
3. Each beak with rounded notch at a right angle to the beak near the tip on the opposing surfaces.
4. Box-jointed, pivot construction.

Use
1. For adjusting the inner and outer arches of face-bows; can handle up to 0.062-inch (1.55-mm) diameter wire.
2. For wire contouring on large-diameter round, oval, or rectangular wires.

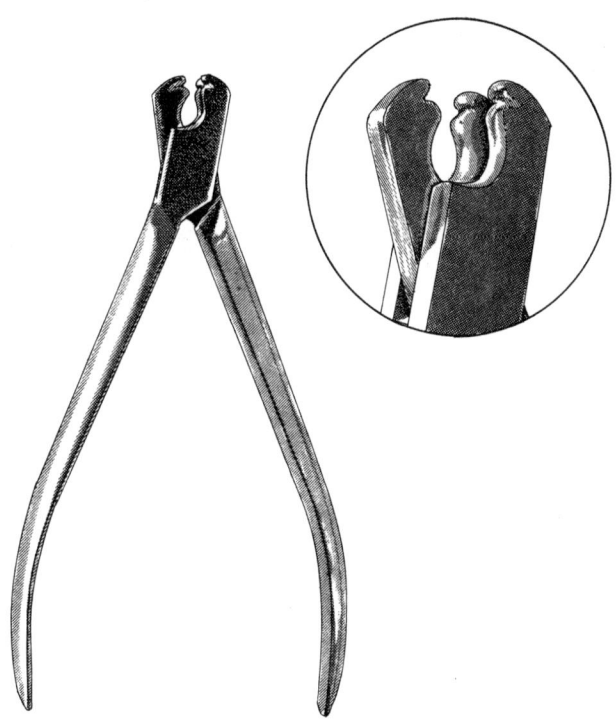

Fig. 8-19

Light-wire pliers (Fig. 8-20)

Physical characteristics
1. Two beaks, with a pyramidal beak opposing a conical one. Pliers varies according to length and taper of the beaks, with the longer-beak pliers more easily forming small-diameter loops.
2. May have grooves at tip of the pyramidal beak opposing the conical beak; these aid in making identical loops and helices and offer a range of sizes.
3. May have cutting edges at the back of the beaks to make it a combination loop-forming pliers and cutter.

Use
1. Mainly to form various loop designs in orthodontic wires, generally light, round wires.
2. To make minor adjustment bends in the archwires.
3. To place metal spring separators.

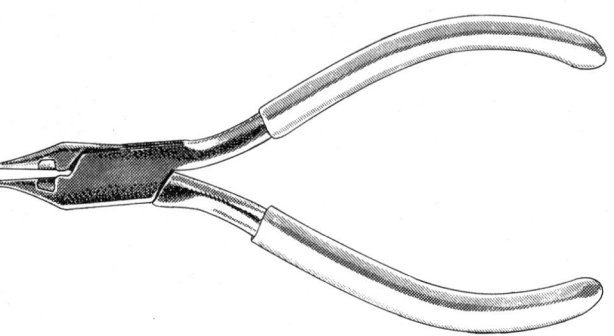

Fig. 8-20

ORTHODONTIC INSTRUMENTS

Arch-forming pliers
(Fig. 8-21)

Physical characteristics
1. Two parallel beaks, with the concave beak fitting around the opposing cylindrical one.
2. The cylindrical beak may have grooves of varying sizes or be nongrooved.
3. Beaks in the long axis of the pliers.

Use
To help form and contour archwires, either round or rectangular, without torquing the wire.

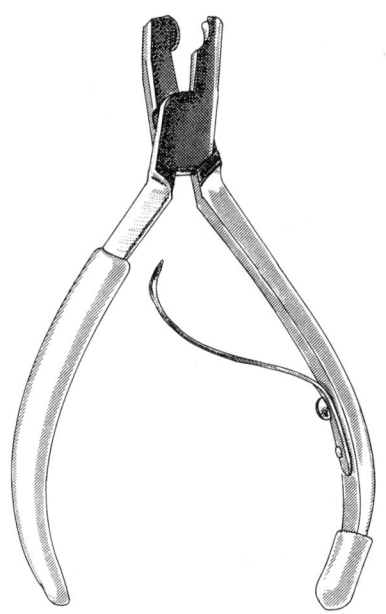

Fig. 8-21

Distal-end–cutting pliers and holder (Fig. 8-22)

Physical characteristics
1. Opposing cutting edges, with beaks at right angles from the long axis of the pliers.
2. Distal to the cutting edges is a safety hold to catch the loose end of the cut archwire.
3. May have adjustable screw joint.
4. Will cut round wires up to 0.020 inch (0.50 mm) in diameter and rectangular wires up to 0.022 × 0.028 inch (0.55 × 0.70 mm).

Use
To cut the distal ends of archwires intraorally; with the safety hold it grips the loose end of the cut archwire, preventing it from becoming embedded in the tissue.

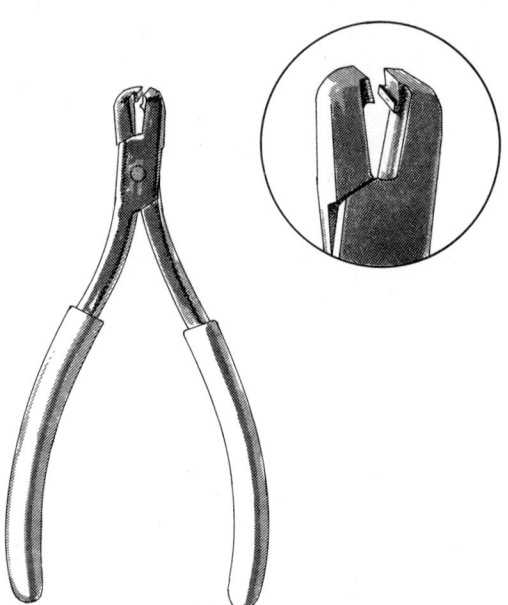

Fig. 8-22

ORTHODONTIC INSTRUMENTS

Weingart utility pliers
(Fig. 8-23)

Physical characteristics
1. Two beaks with opposing serrated tips.
2. The oblong, pointed tips angulated either straight or curved from the long axis of the pliers for a better working angle in making intraoral adjustments.
3. Tips designed close to the center of rotation.
4. Stainless steel construction.
5. May have adjustable screw joint.

Use
For holding or gripping the archwire to make adjustment bends or to place it in and remove it from the mouth.

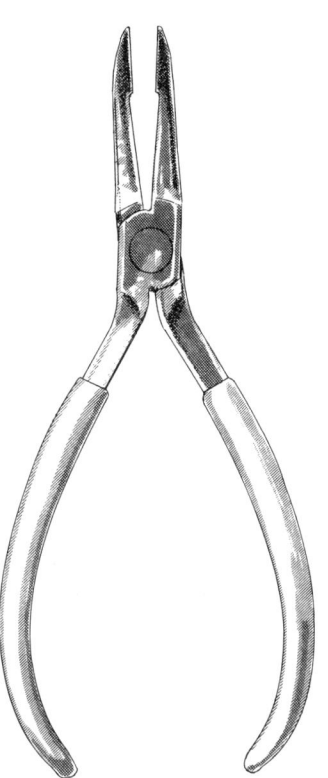

Fig. 8-23

Tweed loop-forming pliers (omega) (Fig. 8-24)

Physical characteristics
1. Two opposing parallel beaks, one concave and one round.
2. The round beak has generally three sections of various diameters, the most common being 0.045, 0.060, and 0.075 inch (1.125, 1.5, and 1.875 mm).
3. Outer one third of concave beak serrated.
4. May have replaceable tips.

Use
To form various loops, especially the omega loop.

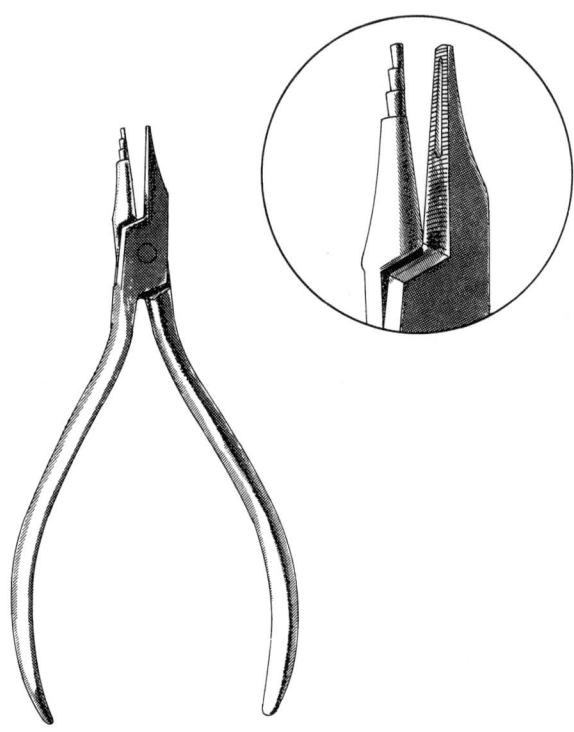

Fig. 8-24

ORTHODONTIC INSTRUMENTS

Ligature pliers (Mathieu style) (Fig. 8-25)

Physical characteristics
1. Positive-locking ratchet and spring in handle for instant opening and closing.
2. Stainless steel construction.
3. Opposing tips serrated and many have serrated tungsten carbide inserts for longer instrument life.
4. Tips vary in length and taper by manufacturer.
5. Pliers available in regular or small.

Use
1. Mainly for tying metal ligature wires.
2. For placing Alastik ligature modules.

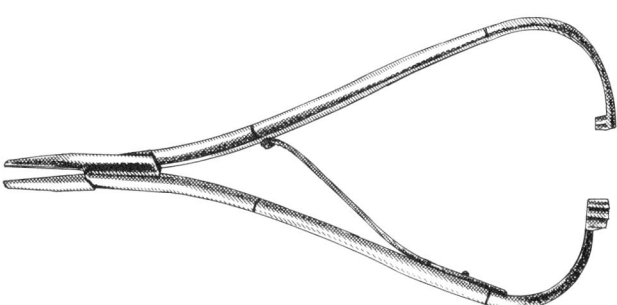

Fig. 8-25

Parallel-action pliers with cutter (Sargent) (Fig. 8-26)

Physical characteristics
1. Heavy-duty pliers with parallel, flat, serrated opposing beaks.
2. Wire cutter on the nonserrated side of one of the beaks.

Use
Mainly for cutting, bending, or holding large-diameter wires in laboratory procedures.

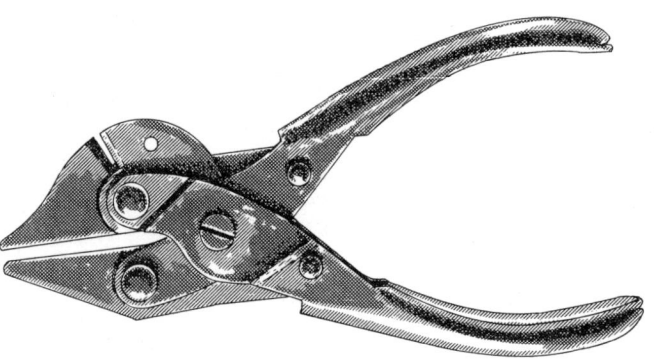

Fig. 8-26

9 PERIODONTAL INSTRUMENTS

Christine P. Klausner
L. H. Klausner

Periodontal instruments are designed to be used in procedures dealing with the identification and treatment of diseases affecting the supporting structures of the teeth—the periodontium. These structures include the gingiva, periodontal ligament, cementum, and alveolar bone. In order to use these instruments effectively, it is important to understand the basic design and function and application of each.

The best way to identify periodontal instruments is to classify them according to the functions they perform. The following list groups the instruments into categories as they are used for specific procedures:
1. Examination instruments
2. Scaling instruments
3. Cleansing and polishing instruments
4. Periodontal surgical instruments
5. Electrosurgical instruments

EXAMINATION INSTRUMENTS

All dental treatment begins with an assessment of the conditions existing in the patient's mouth. A thorough tactile and visual examination is best accomplished by using the proper instruments—a mouth mirror, explorer, and periodontal probe.

Mouth mirror (see Figs. 2-2 and 2-3)

Use
1. To retract the cheek or tongue.
2. To provide indirect vision.
3. To provide indirect illumination.

Explorers (see Fig. 2-1)

Use
1. To detect tooth surface irregularities and dental deposits.
2. To check tooth or restoration smoothness following instrumentation.
3. To detect dental caries.

Periodontal probe

Physical characteristics
1. Tapered, rodlike blade with a blunt, rounded tip calibrated at 1 to 3 mm intervals.
2. Thin blades with angled shanks to allow easy insertion into a pocket.
3. Some probes color-banded to indicate millimeter markings (Fig. 9-1, A to C).

Use
1. To locate and measure the depth of periodontal pockets.
2. To determine pocket configuration.
3. To locate calculus and identify tooth surface irregularities.

Application (Fig. 9-1, D)
1. In measuring a pocket, blade of the probe aligned parallel to the long axis of the tooth within the sulcus and positioned at the epithelial attachment.
2. Several measurements made on each tooth to determine pocket depth and configurations.
3. A normal sulcus depth considered to be up to 3 mm.

PERIODONTAL INSTRUMENTS

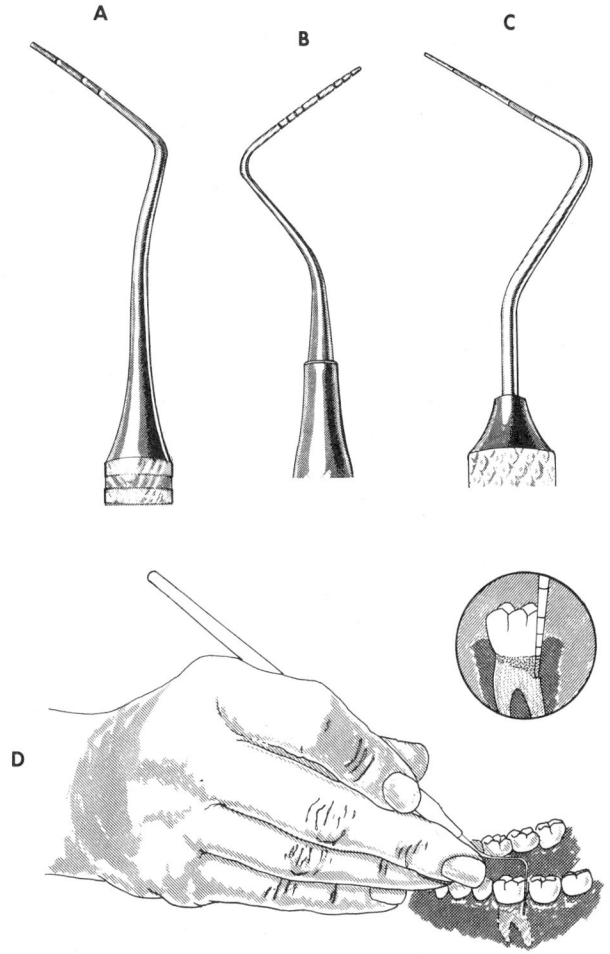

Fig. 9-1

121

SCALING INSTRUMENTS These instruments are designed to remove dental deposits from tooth surfaces and to smooth the tooth so it will resist reaccumulation of these deposits. Depending on the design and shape of the instrument and the gingival tissue adaptation, the scaler may be used supragingivally or subgingivally for heavy or fine deposits.

Sickle scaler

Physical characteristics
1. Blade triangular in cross section, with two cutting edges that converge to form a point. Cutting edges formed by the junction of the two lateral surfaces with the inner surface (face) of the blade.
2. Blade design limits subgingival insertion depending on the health of the gingiva (Fig. 9-2, *B*).
3. Anterior sickle designed with the blade in the same plane as the shank.
4. Posterior sickles (also known as jacquettes) are paired instruments with various angulated shanks to allow access to all tooth surfaces of posterior teeth.
5. Available in a variety of blade sizes and shank types to adapt to specific uses.
6. Fig. 9-2 illustrates *A*, curved and straight sickles and *C*, paired jacquettes.

Use
To remove calculus located supragingivally or slightly below the gingival margin when access is possible.

Application (Fig. 9-2, *B* and *D*)
1. For instrument placement in calculus removal, blade positioned apical to the deposit with the side of the tip of the cutting edge contacting the tooth surface.
2. A short, coronal pull stroke directed in line with the long axis of the tooth.

PERIODONTAL INSTRUMENTS

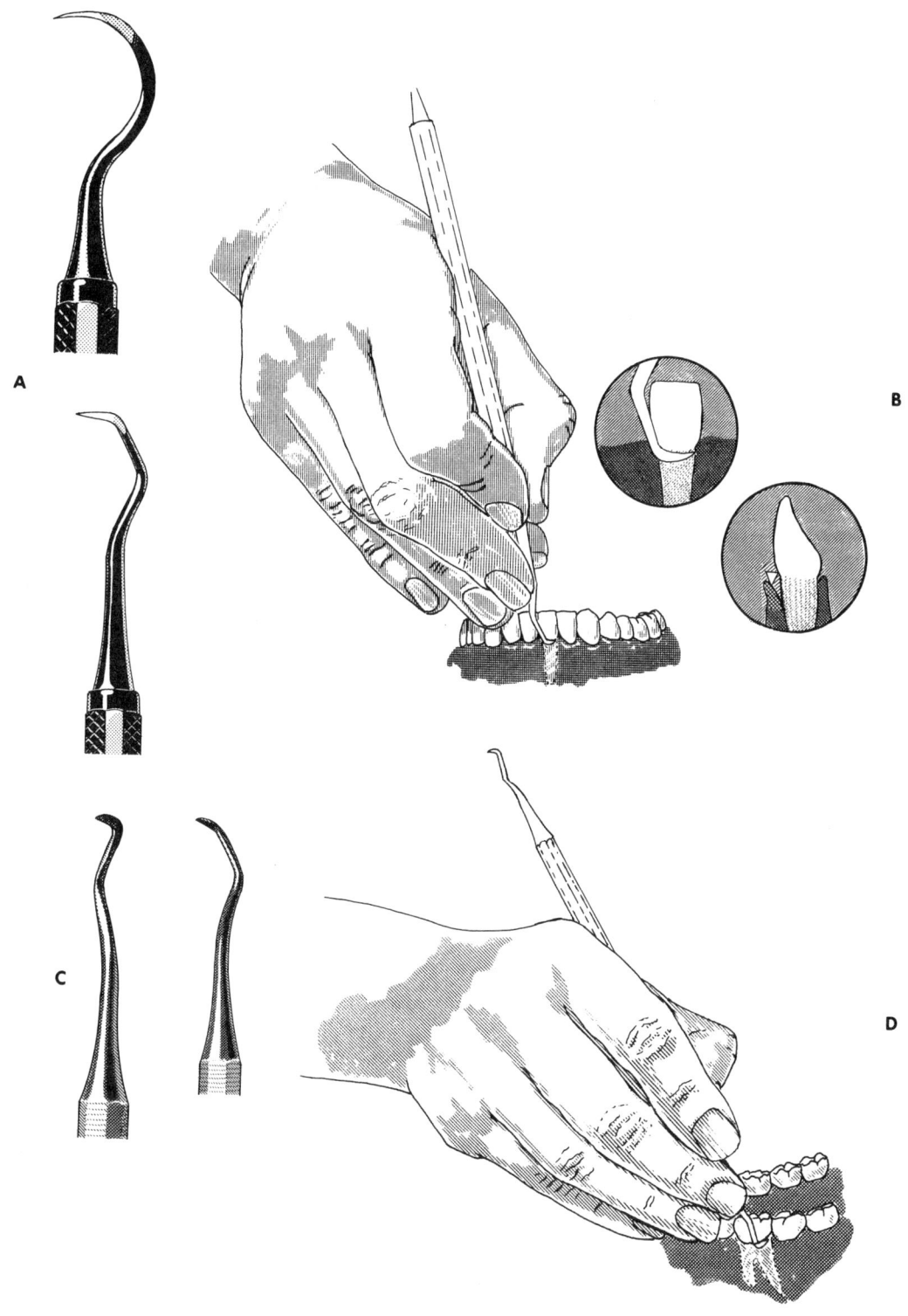

Fig. 9-2

Chisel scaler

Physical characteristics
1. Working end consists of a straight cutting edge with a flat, wedge-shaped blade beveled at a 45-degree angle.
2. Blade, shank, and handle continuous, with a slight curvature in the shank (Fig. 9-3, *A*).

Use
To remove supragingival calculus from proximal surfaces of anterior teeth.

Application (Fig. 9-3, *B*)
1. Application restricted to proximal surfaces of anterior teeth where interdental gingiva is missing.
2. Cutting edge positioned parallel to the long axis of the tooth on a proximal tooth surface with the entire edge contacting tooth.
3. Push stroke used in a horizontal direction, moving in a labiolingual direction.

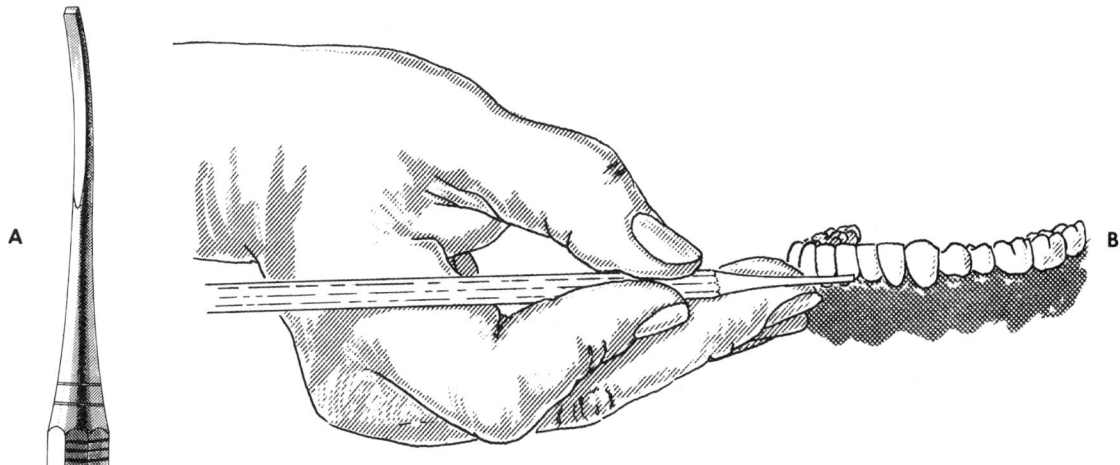

Fig. 9-3

PERIODONTAL INSTRUMENTS

Hoe scaler

Physical characteristics

1. Blade shape similar to a garden hoe, with a straight, single cutting edge beveled at 45 degrees.
2. Blade angulated to the shank at about 100 degrees.
3. Shanks either angled or curved.
4. Two pairs required for access to all tooth surfaces—one pair for posterior scaling (Fig. 9-4, *A* and *B*) and one pair for anterior scaling (Fig. 9-4, *C* and *D*).

Use

To remove large, accessible calculus deposits located supragingivally or slightly below the gingival margin if the tissue is easily displaced.

Application

1. A two-point contact of the blade and the shank on the tooth maintained for stability.
2. Shank parallel to the long axis of the tooth and a pull stroke in a coronal direction employed for calculus removal.

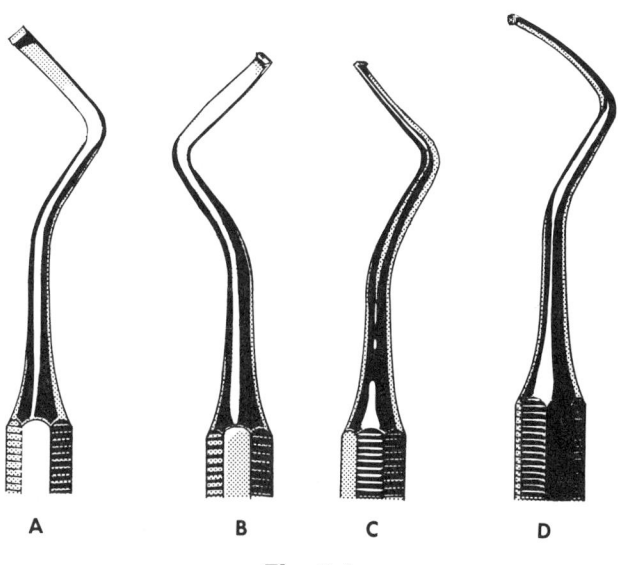

Fig. 9-4

File scaler

Physical characteristics
1. Series of hoelike cutting edges aligned close together and beveled at 90 to 105 degrees on the blade surface.
2. Length of the cutting edges are shorter than that of the hoe, accommodating subgingival application.
3. Like the hoe, files come in two pairs with curved or angled shanks (Fig. 9-5, *A* to *D*).

Use
1. To remove tenacious deposits of calculus located on the tooth, supragingivally and subgingivally.
2. To smooth the cementoenamel junction of the tooth.
3. To smooth overextended amalgam restorations.

Application (Fig. 9-5, *E*)
1. May be adapted either subgingivally or supragingivally.
2. Entire blade surface placed on the affected area, with the shank parallel to the long axis of the tooth.
3. A pull stroke used in a coronal direction.

PERIODONTAL INSTRUMENTS

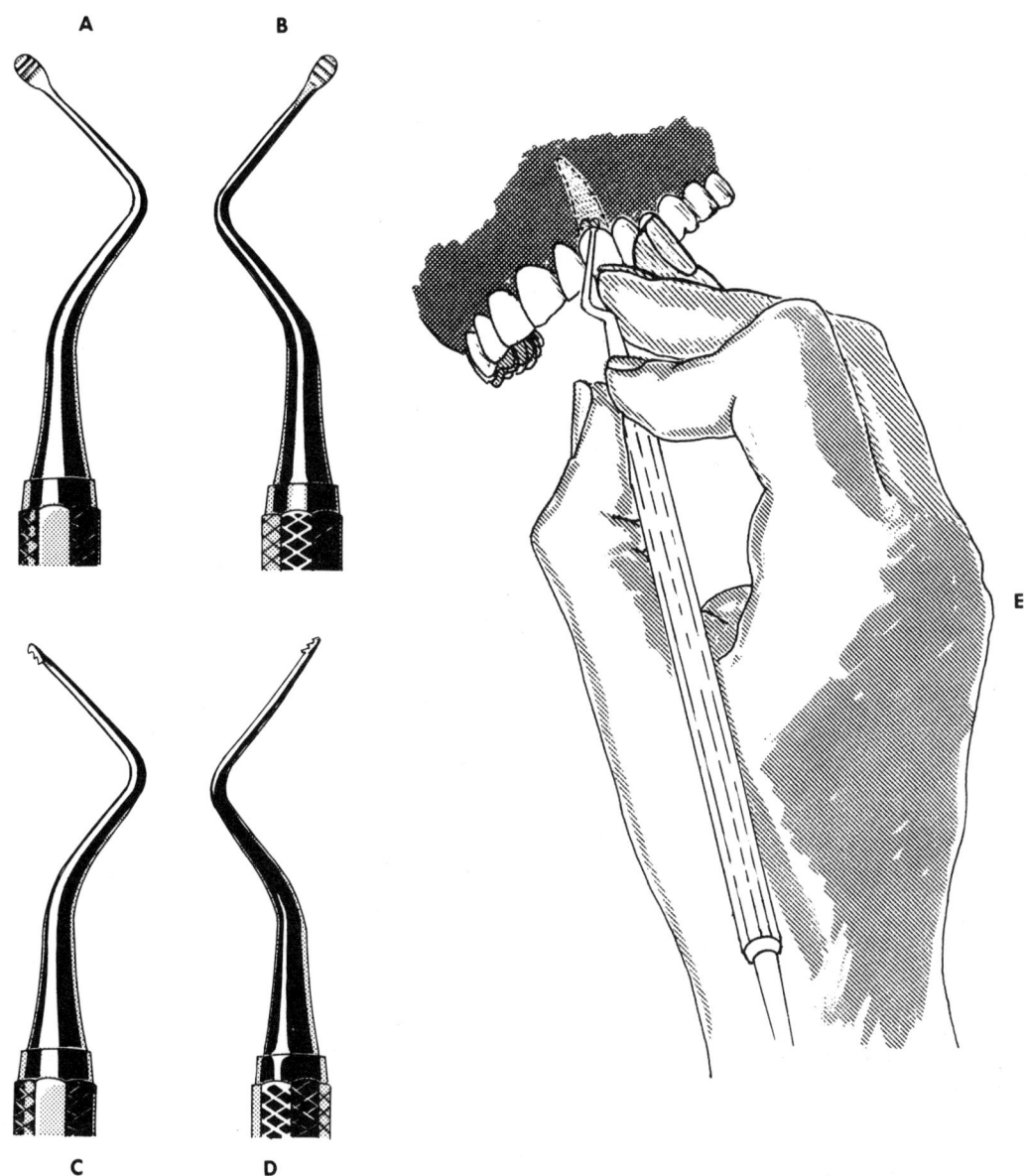

Fig. 9-5

Curettes

Physical characteristics
1. Spoon-shaped blade, with one continuous cutting edge forming a rounded tip; in cross section the blade shape resembles a semicircle, with the face and lateral sides meeting to form the cutting edge (Fig. 9-6).
2. Anterior curettes designed with blades and shanks in the same plane.
3. Posterior curettes characterized by shanks of various lengths and angulation.
4. Curved, rounded configuration allows the blade to adapt well to tooth surfaces and minimizes tissue trauma.
5. Two basic blade designs: the universal and the specific.
6. Universal curette: a paired instrument designed to adapt to most areas of the dentition, by modifying hand and finger positioning; blade characterized by two parallel cutting edges that form a rounded tip, such as the Columbia 13/14 (Fig. 9-6, *A* and *B*).
7. Specific curettes: a set of several instruments that adapt to specific anatomic areas of the teeth, with only one lateral cutting edge used for instrumentation. Blade curvature and shank angulation limit the use of each curette in the set to particular tooth surfaces. The Gracey curettes are representative of this type and are well suited for subgingival scaling and root planing (Fig. 9-6, *C* to *F*).

Use
1. To remove supragingival and subgingival dental deposits.
2. To smooth root surfaces (root plane).
3. To remove the soft tissue lining of a periodontal pocket (gingival curettage).
4. To fine scale and smooth tooth surfaces after the use of other scalers.

Application
1. Universal curette used with a pull stroke, while the specific curette used with a push or pull stroke.
2. Blade placed at the base of the periodontal pocket or apical to the dental deposit.
3. In a root-planning procedure the cementum is smoothed.
4. During curettage, the cutting edge removes the soft tissue lining of the pocket wall.
5. Used in a vertical, horizontal, or oblique direction.

PERIODONTAL INSTRUMENTS

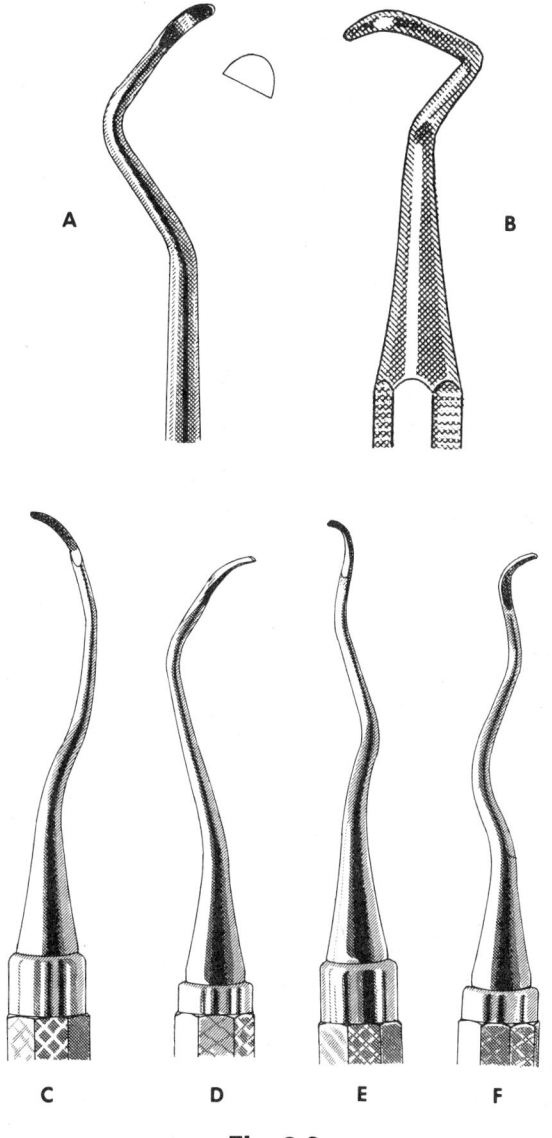

Fig. 9-6

Ultrasonic scaling device

Physical characteristics
1. Consists of an electronic control unit, a handpiece, a set of interchangeable scaling tips, and a foot control (Fig. 9-7, *A* and *B*).
2. Mode of action based on the principle of converting high-frequency sound waves into mechanical energy, which creates rapid vibrations of the scaling tip.
3. Different models produce varying tip vibration patterns.
4. In periodontal instrumentation, an ultrasonic scaler may produce 25,000 vibrations per second, with a stroke length of about 0.0004 inch (0.001 cm).
5. Deposits on the tooth fractured off by the vibrating motion.
6. Heat generated by these vibrations can damage gingival and tooth tissues, so a water spray cooling system is contained in the unit. Spray directed toward the end of the tip to help dissipate the heat and rinse away the debris.

Use
To dislodge calculus, stain, and soft debris from tooth surfaces using ultrasonic vibrations and water; generally used supragingivally.

Application
1. Applied with light pressure, using short, rapid, vertical or oblique strokes.
2. Tip kept in constant motion and must contact the deposit to dislodge it.
3. Improper use may produce roughening, scratching, or gouging of the root surfaces.
4. Instrumentation with the curette should follow all ultrasonic scaling to smooth the tooth surface.

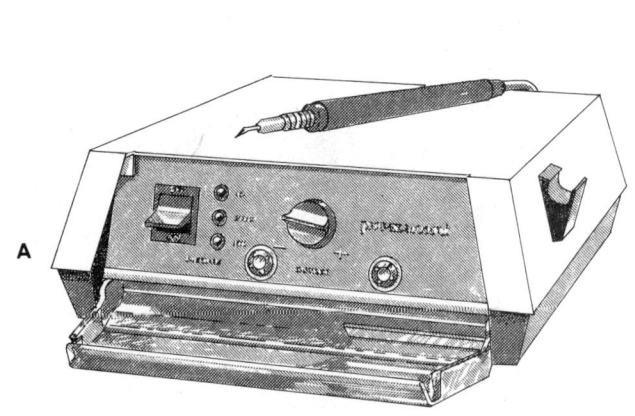
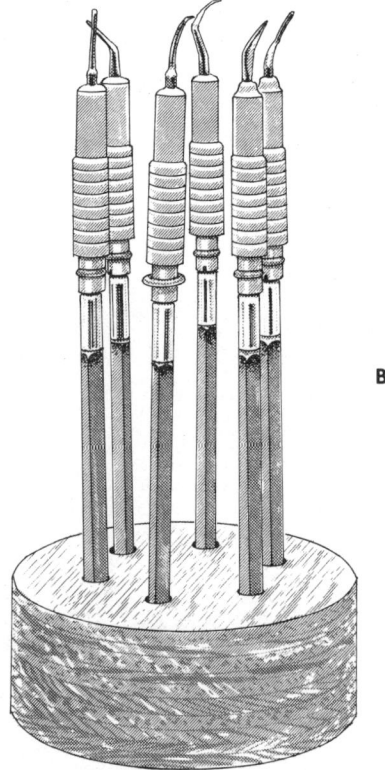

Fig. 9-7

PERIODONTAL INSTRUMENTS

CLEANSING AND POLISHING INSTRUMENTS

Once the removal of stain and calculus has been accomplished by scaling and root-planing procedures, the teeth are cleansed and polished before topical fluoride is applied. Cleansing and polishing involves the use of mechanical and hand instruments for the removal of soft films and plaque from the crowns and exposed root surfaces of the teeth. This cleansing and polishing procedure creates a very smooth and shiny surface that resists reaccumulation of oral debris and plaque. Smooth surfaces assist patients with their oral hygiene maintenance.

Mechanical polishing instruments

PROPHYLAXIS ANGLE
Physical characteristics
1. Rotary instrument that attaches to a dental handpiece.
2. Either right-angled or contra-angled in design.
3. Fig. 9-8 illustrates the latch, snap-on, and screw-type head designs.

Use
To accept mechanical polishing attachments such as rubber cups and bristle brushes.

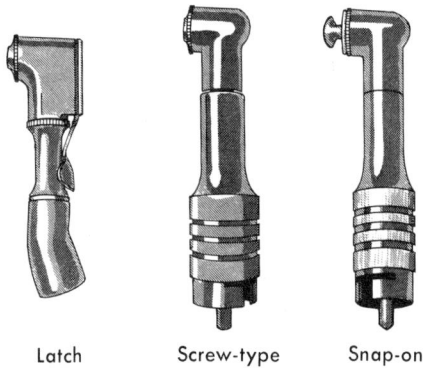

Latch   Screw-type   Snap-on

Fig. 9-8

RUBBER POLISHING CUP (Fig. 9-9, A, top and bottom)

Physical characteristics

1. Ribbed (top) or webbed (bottom) internal configurations.
2. Natural or synthetic rubber.
3. Soft to firm texture.
4. Variety of sizes and shapes.
5. Attachment styles—screw, latch, or snap-on.

Use

To carry and place polishing paste on tooth surfaces. When power activates the prophylaxis angle, the polishing cup rotates to clean and smooth the tooth.

BRISTLE BRUSHES (Fig. 9-9, A, middle)

Physical characteristics

1. Natural or synthetic bristles.
2. Cup or wheel shapes.
3. Various sizes.
4. Tapered or flat bristles.
5. Attachment styles—screw, latch, or snap-on.

Use

This attachment cleans pits and fissures and other tooth surface irregularities that may harbor plaque not removed by the rubber polishing cup.

Application (Fig. 9-9, B)

1. The rubber cup is filled with polishing paste and applied to the tooth.
2. After paste applied to several teeth, the handpiece is started.
3. Light, intermittent pressure used to clean and polish the tooth surface.

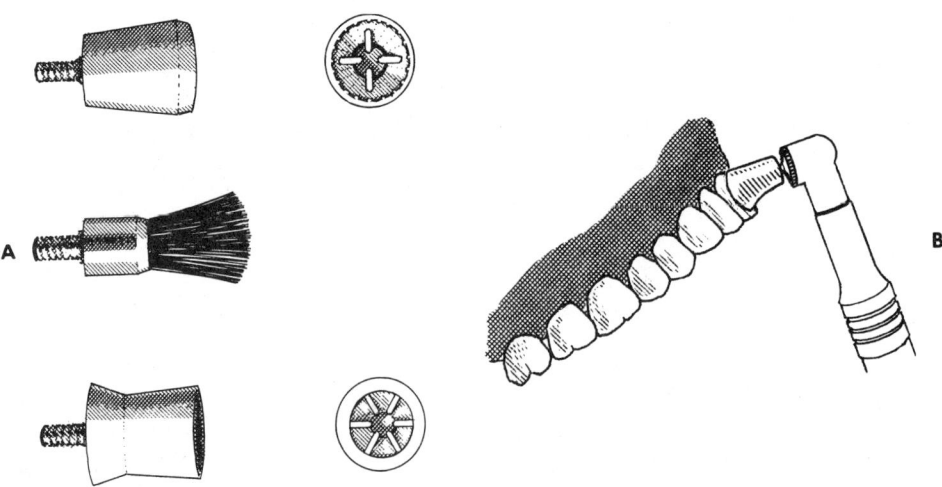

Fig. 9-9

PERIODONTAL INSTRUMENTS

Manual polishing instruments

PORTE POLISHER
Physical characteristics
1. Two common designs available: the Ivory porte polisher and the Mynol porte polisher.
2. Ivory porte polisher a single-ended instrument with a straight or contra-angled shank.
3. Mynol porte polisher a double-ended instrument with angle variations of the shank for access to various tooth surfaces (Fig. 9-10).
4. The wood points generally made from orangewood and beveled on the working end; orangewood hard enough to resist the pressure of polishing without fracturing, yet porous enough to hold polishing agents.

Use
To remove plaque and oral debris from tooth surfaces with the inserted wood points. It has the advantage of adapting to surfaces inaccessible with the prophylaxis angle and can be used on exposed root surfaces that may be hypersensitive.

Application
1. The wood point inserted into a small mounting hole at the end of the porte polisher.
2. A small amount of polishing agent accumulated on the wood point and placed on the tooth.
3. A short, burnishing stroke used to remove soft deposits and polish the tooth.

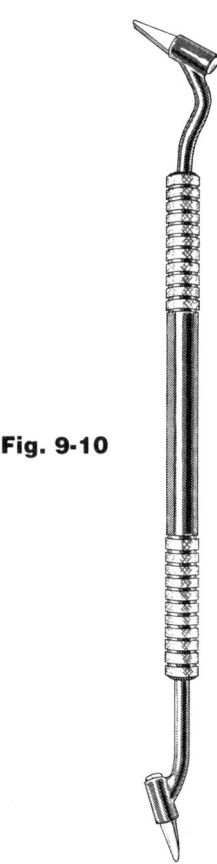

Fig. 9-10

ORANGEWOOD STICK

Although not a commonly used instrument, the orangewood stick demonstrates the same principle as the porte polisher. It is a straight stick with a beveled end. Its use is limited because of problems of adapting the working end to some tooth surfaces.

DENTAL FLOSS OR TAPE
Physical characteristics
1. Dental floss: threadlike material used on proximal tooth surfaces.
2. Dental tape: ribbonlike material.
3. Available in waxed and unwaxed types. The unwaxed product recommended if fluoride is to be applied to the dentition, because a waxed coating may be left by the waxed tape or floss and may inhibit fluoride penetration to the tooth.

Use
To polish the proximal surfaces of teeth inaccessible to other polishing instruments.

Application (Fig. 9-11)
1. With fingers stabilized on the dentition, the floss or tape is passed through the proximal contacts with a gentle sawing motion.
2. Each proximal tooth surface polished by wrapping the floss or tape in a C-shaped configuration around the tooth and using an up-and-down stroke.
3. Care must be taken not to traumatize the gingival tissue but to guide the floss or tape into the sulcus area.
4. Removal accomplished by using a sawing motion or by drawing the floss or tape from under the contact.

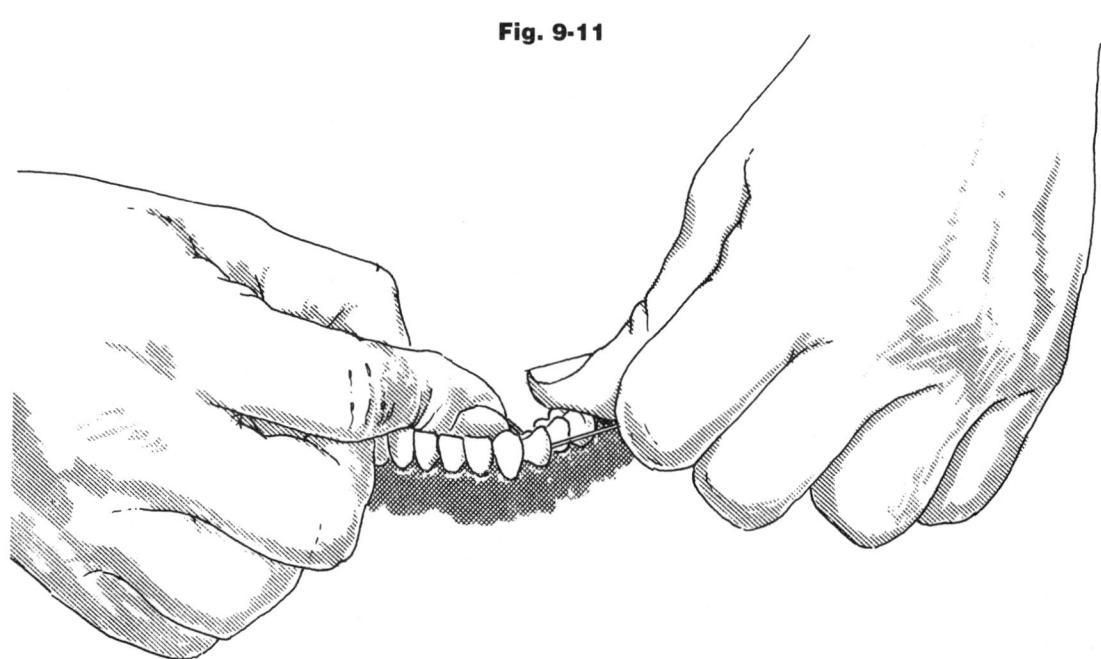

Fig. 9-11

PERIODONTAL INSTRUMENTS

POLISHING STRIPS

Physical characteristics

1. Thin, flexible tapes of linen or plastic impregnated with abrasive particles.
2. A variety of abrasives available.
3. Also known as linen abrasive strips or finishing strips.

Use

To remove stain from proximal tooth surfaces when other techniques unsuccessful.

Application (Fig. 9-12)

1. May be introduced through the contact (using an area of the strip that does not have abrasive) or may be threaded below the contact area.
2. Strip wrapped around the tooth in a C-shaped manner and short, back-and-forth strokes used, forcing the abrasive particles onto the stained surface.
3. Care must be taken not to traumatize the gingival tissue or open the proximal contact.
4. This procedure followed by polishing with dental floss or tape to remove excess abrasive particles.

POLISHING AGENTS

Abrasive pastes or powders are used to remove soft deposits and to smooth tooth surfaces. The pastes are commercially prepared and available in coarse to fine textures. They may be flavored and may contain fluoride. The powders are also available in varying textures. The type of powder used will influence the abrasive action of the agent. Silex, pumice, zirconium silicate, and tin oxide are commonly used powders. They are prepared by adding water, glycerin, or mouth-wash to form a slurry that is applied to the tooth.

Fig. 9-12

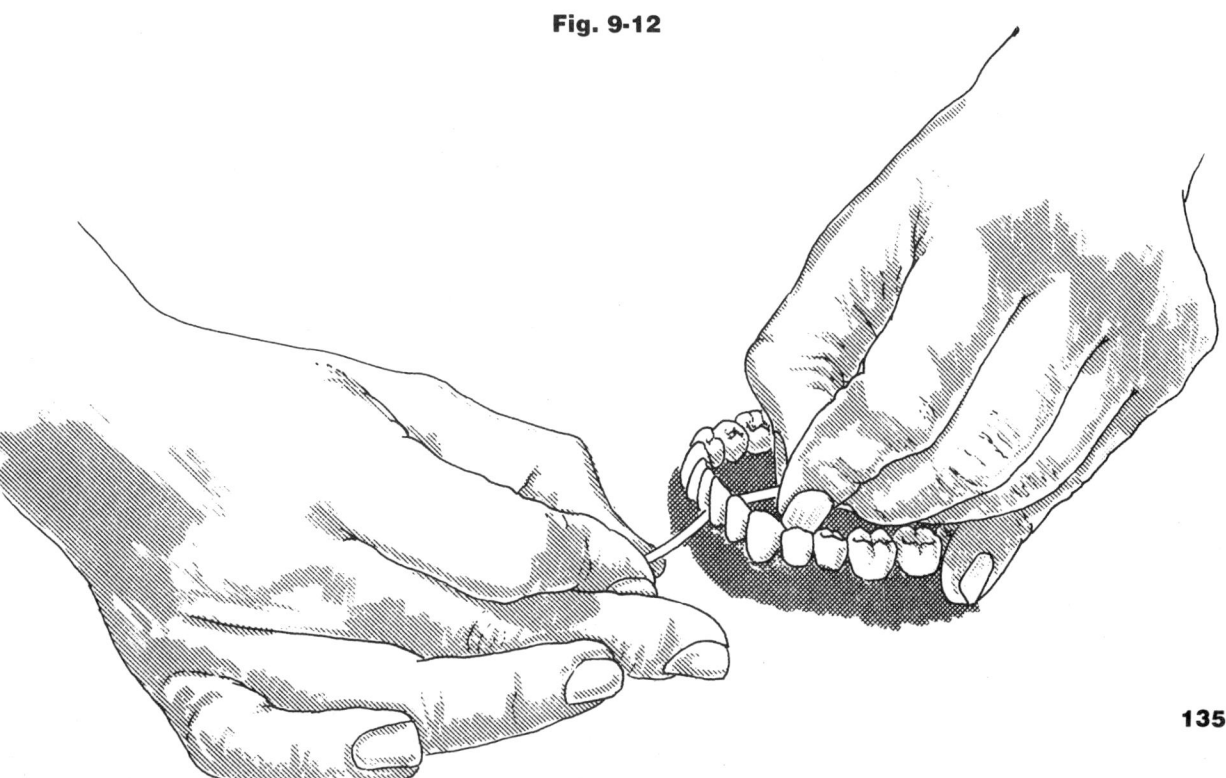

PERIODONTAL SURGICAL INSTRUMENTS

Surgical procedures in the treatment of periodontal disease are used to correct deformities of the periodontium that may contribute to the progression of the disease. The most frequent indications for periodontal surgery are gingival or periodontal pocket depths that inhibit effective oral hygiene. This may involve surgical reduction or recontouring of soft (gingival) and hard (osseous) tissues.

Soft-tissue surgical instruments

PERIODONTAL POCKET MARKER

Physical characteristics
1. Similar in shape to cotton pliers.
2. Comes as a paired set.
3. Working end consists of a sharp tip bent at a right angle and an opposing blunt tip slightly bowed to conform to the contour of a tooth (Fig. 9-13, A).

Use
1. To identify pocket depths on the facial or lingual aspects of gingival tissue by producing external bleeding points.
2. To serve as a guide for incision placement during surgical procedures.

Application (Fig. 9-13, B)
1. Pocket marking accomplished by inserting the blunt end of the instrument to the bottom of a pocket and aligning it with the long axis of the tooth.
2. Pressure exerted to close the ends together, producing a bleeding point on the external surface of the gingiva.
3. Several markings made to indicate the course of the pocket.

PERIODONTAL INSTRUMENTS

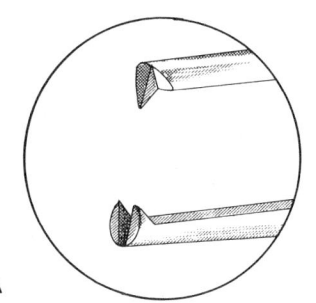

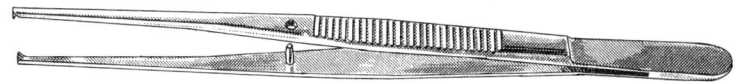

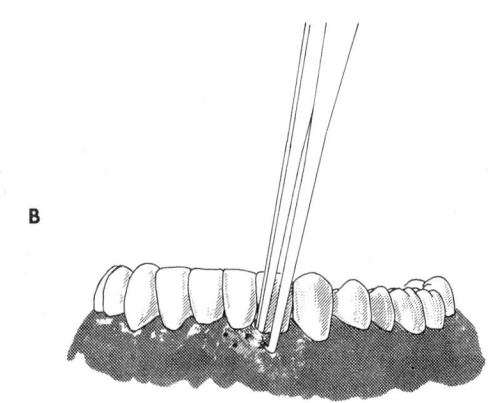

Fig. 9-13

PERIODONTAL KNIVES
Physical characteristics
1. Paired instruments with angled shanks for ease of adaptation.
2. Thin, flattened blades come in a variety of shapes.
3. Entire periphery of the blade sharpened to accommodate the use of a push or pull slicing motion (Fig. 9-14, *A* and *B*).

Use
1. To make various types of incisions, especially those involving removal or recontouring of soft tissues.
2. To free interproximal tissue after the initial incisions.
3. To thin or scallop flaps.

Application
Depends on the specific surgical procedure being performed; for example, Fig. 9-14, *C* shows the technique of incising gingival tissue.

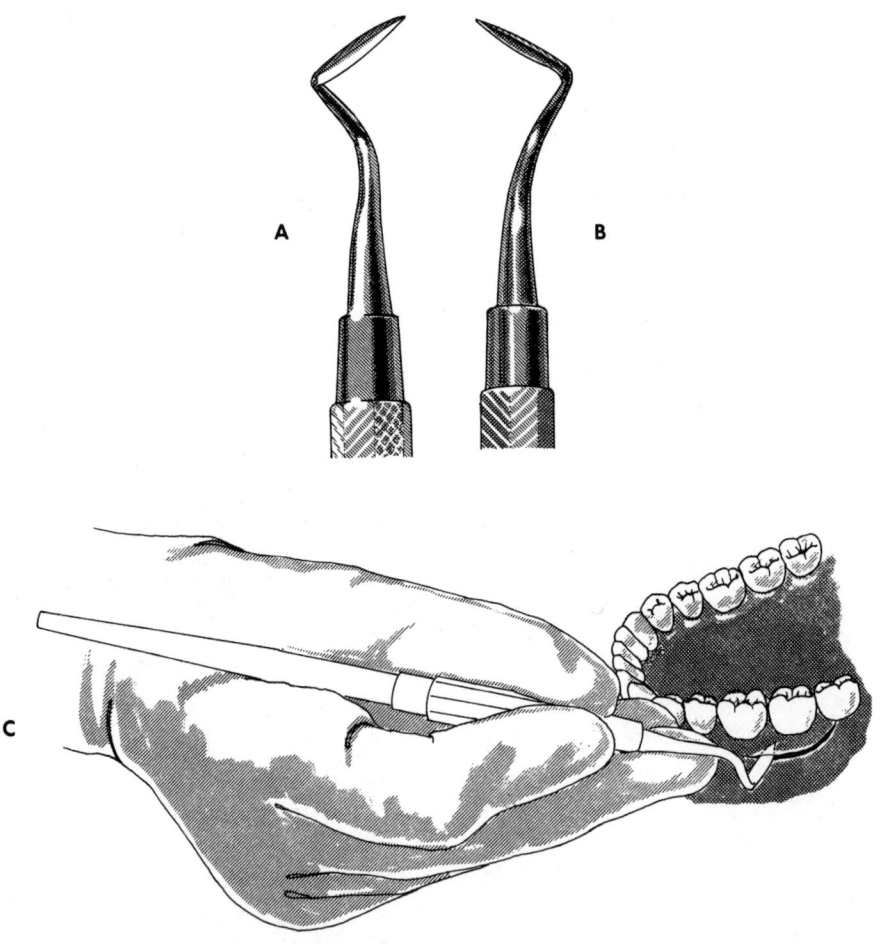

Fig. 9-14

PERIODONTAL INSTRUMENTS

PERIOSTEAL ELEVATOR

Physical characteristics

1. Double-ended instrument.
2. Blade shapes include a rounded or straight cutting edge or a sharp point.
3. Working ends may be of graduated size and characterized by a slight convexity.
4. Blade, shank, and handle aligned in the same plane (Fig. 9-15, *A*).

Use

For reflection and retraction of the mucoperiosteum after initial incisions of the gingival tissue have been made.

Application (Fig. 9-15, *B*)

1. The blade portion separates soft tissue from bone, with the convex side of the blade against the soft tissue; this reduces the tendency for tearing and puncturing of gingiva.
2. Tissue reflection accomplished with push and prying strokes.

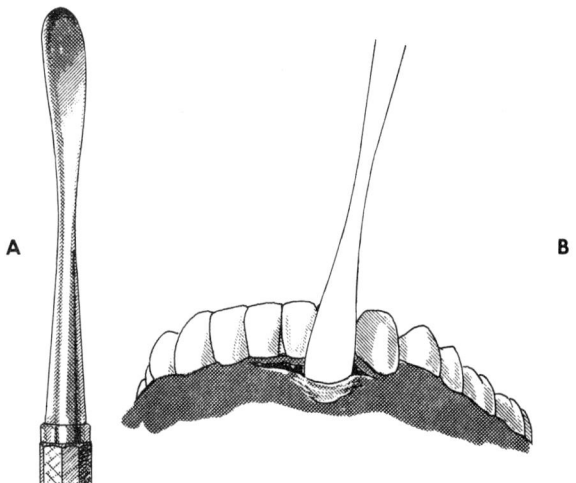

Fig. 9-15

SURGICAL SCISSORS

Physical characteristics
1. Available in a variety of styles, with choice depending on individual preference and particular use.
2. Fig. 9-16 illustrates *A*, straight, *B*, curved, and *C*, angled scissors.
3. Smooth or serrated blades.
4. Blunt or pointed tips.
5. Available in various sizes.

Use
For enlarging initial incisions, trimming tissue, incising muscle attachments and frenectomies, and cutting suture material.

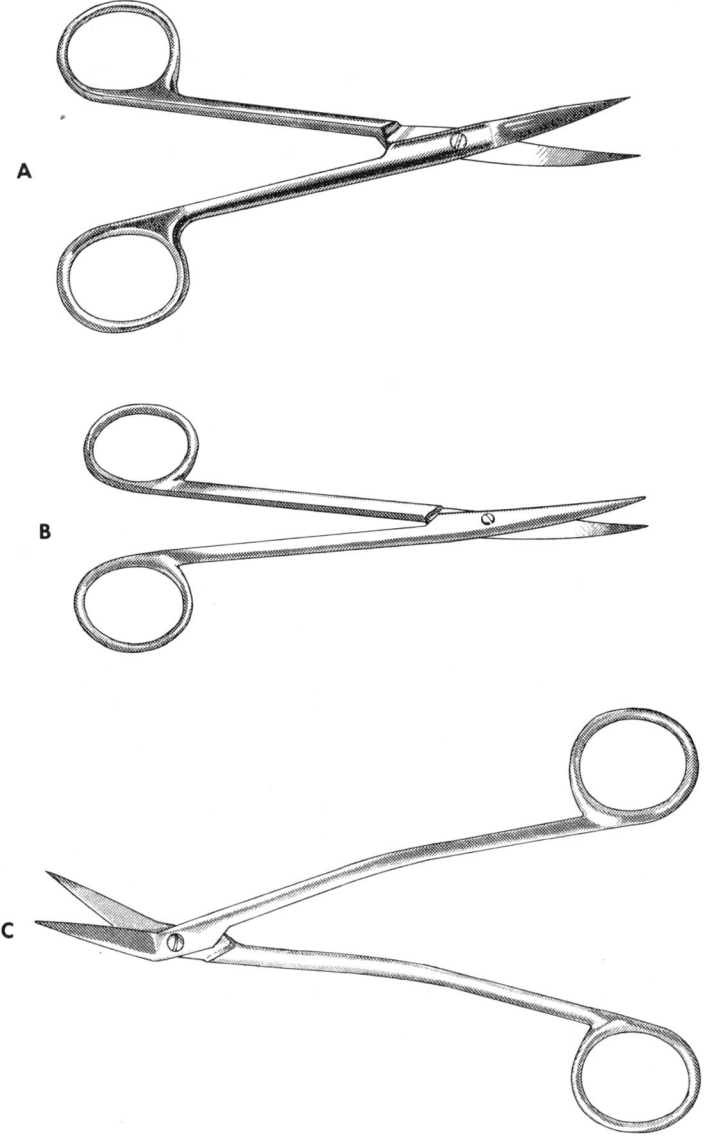

Fig. 9-16

PERIODONTAL INSTRUMENTS

SURGICAL CURETTES AND SICKLES

Physical characteristics
1. Similar to scaling and root planning instruments.
2. Blade and shank design is wider and heavier for surgical procedures.
3. Fig. 9-17 illustrates curettes (*A* to *C*) and sickles (*D* and *E*).

Use
For removal of hard deposits, granulation tissue, and fibrous interdental tissue.

Application (Fig. 9-17, *F*)
Same technique as scaling and root planing.

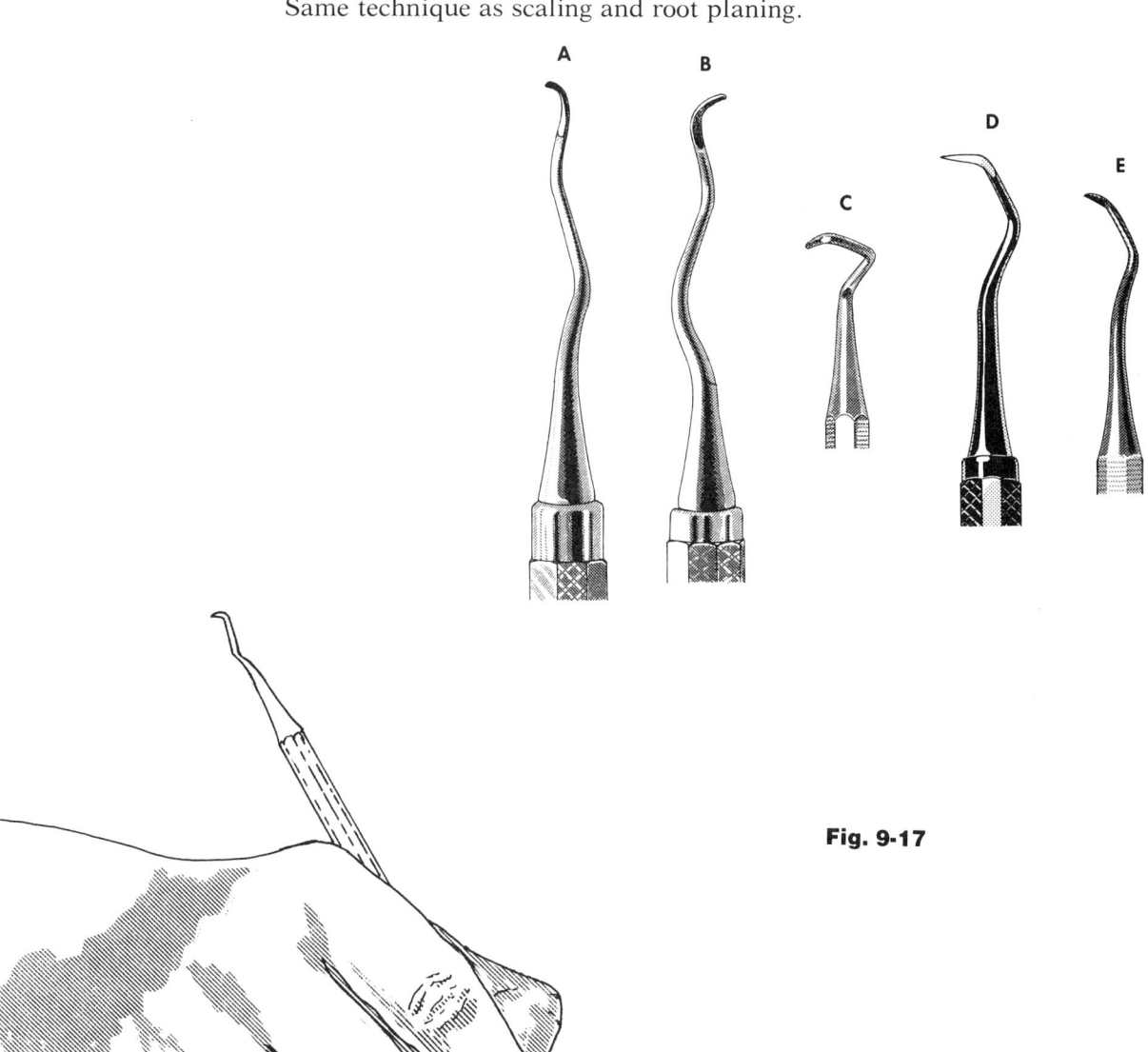

Fig. 9-17

141

SCALPELS

Physical characteristics
1. Sterile, disposable blades (Fig. 9-18, *A*); attach to a handle (Fig. 9-18, *B*).
2. Most common styles are (Fig. 9-18, *A*):

    No. 15—traditionally shaped surgical blade for general use

    No. 11—long, pointed blade with one cutting edge, useful for delicate sulcular incisions

    No. 12 and no. 12B—"hawk-billed" blades, for making incisions at the gingival tissue margins and following the contours of the teeth; no. 12 sharp only on the inner surface of the curve and no. 12B sharp on both inner and outer surfaces

Use
For flap, mucogingival, and graft operations, gingivoplasty, and gingivectomies.

Application (Fig. 9-18, C)
1. Blades designed with one cutting edge used with a push or pull motion.
2. No. 12B blade with two cutting edges accommodates a push or pull stroke.

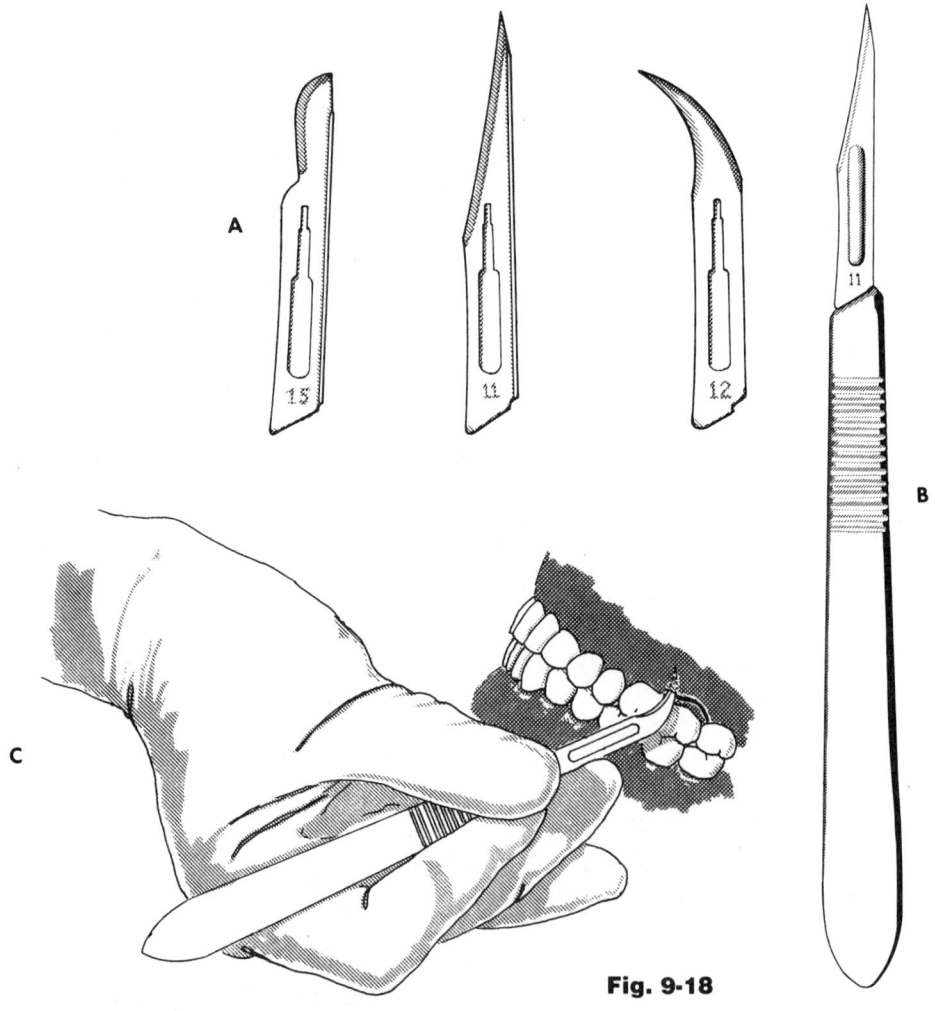

Fig. 9-18

Hard-tissue surgical instruments

SURGICAL CHISELS AND HOES
Physical characteristics
1. Similar to scaling instruments but with heavier shank and blade.
2. Fig. 9-19 illustrates a surgical chisel.

Use
For removing and reshaping bone after soft-tissue reflection.

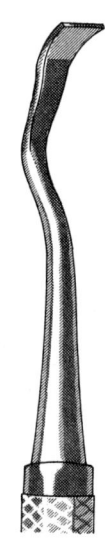

Fig. 9-19

RONGEURS

Physical characteristics
1. Resembles a forceps.
2. Two styles include a side-cutting rongeur and an end-biting rongeur.
3. Either large or small sizes (Fig. 9-20, *A* and *B*).

Use
For trimming alveolar bone.

Application (Fig. 9-20, *C*)
Nipping action recontours alveolar bone.

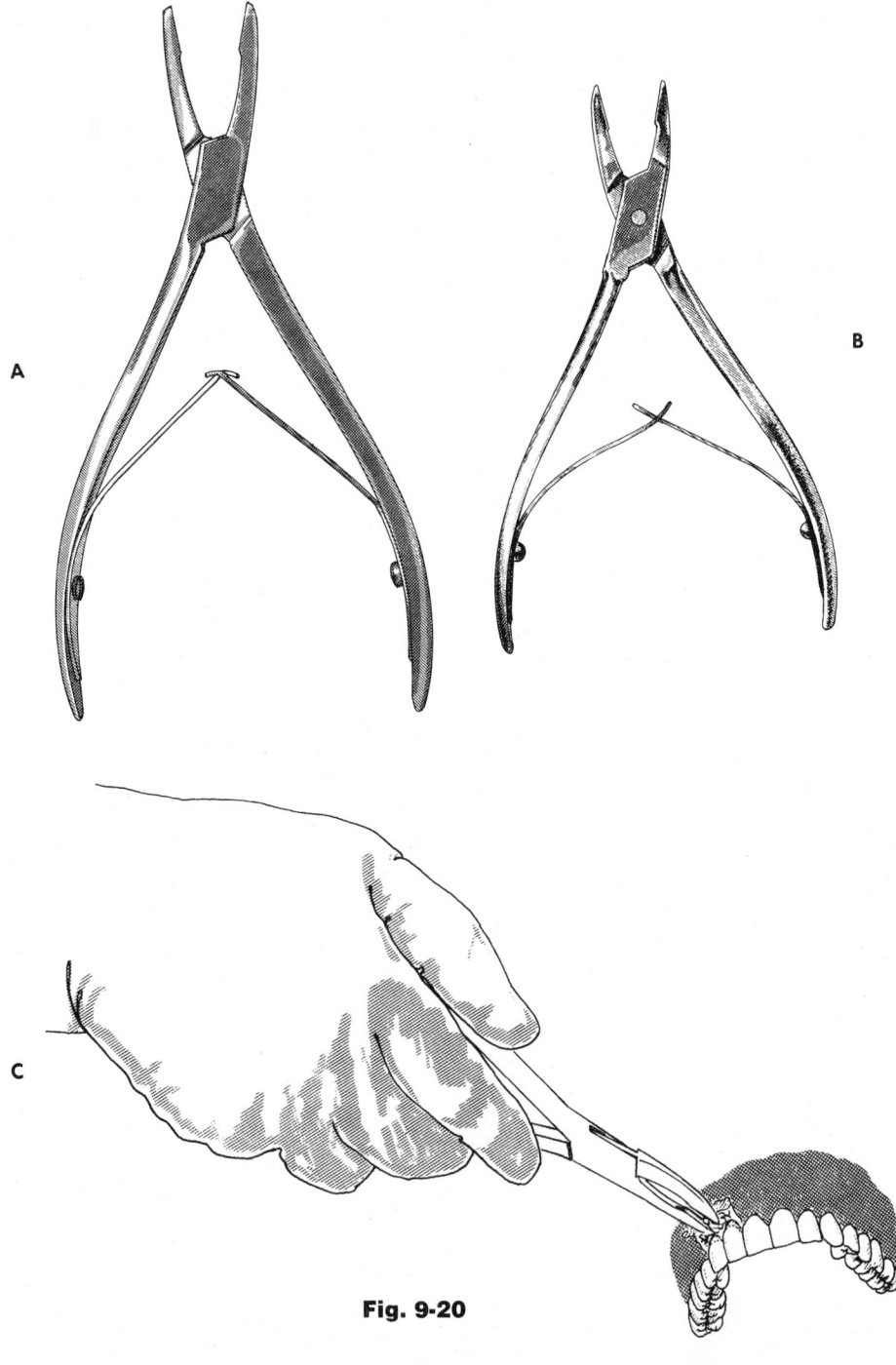

Fig. 9-20

PERIODONTAL INSTRUMENTS

BONE FILES

Physical characteristics
1. Available in two types.
2. The first similar in design to scaling file but wider and heavier; used with a pull stroke.
3. The second an interdental file that has a rod-shaped working end with a series of closely aligned blades along the length of the rod; used with a pull stroke (Fig. 9-21, *A*).

Use
1. For minor bone removal.
2. For smoothing rough ledges (spicules) of bone.

Application
Fig. 9-21, *B* demonstrates use of an interdental file.

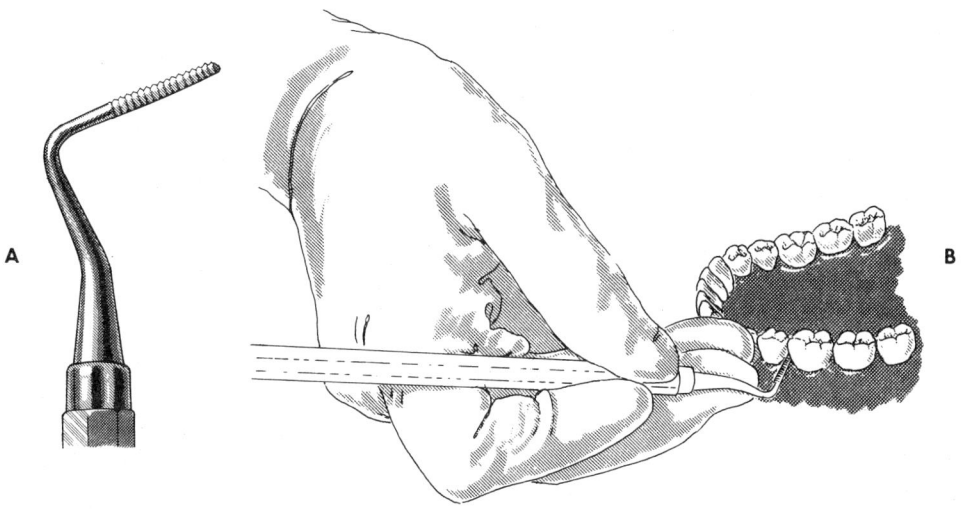

Fig. 9-21

ROTATING INSTRUMENTS
A selection of diamonds and burs is available to be used with slow- and high-seed handpieces (Chapter 5) for minor bone recontouring.

ELECTROSURGICAL INSTRUMENTS

Physical characteristics

1. Unit consists of a control box, foot and/or hand control, and two terminals (Fig. 9-22, *A*).
2. One terminal grounded to the patient; the other holds the electrosurgical handpiece.
3. The tip incises soft tissue in response to current flow activated by the foot control.
4. Various probe tip styles available (Fig. 9-22, *B*).

Use

To recontour soft tissue by employing an arc of electric current. This technique cauterizes small blood vessels to limit hemorrhaging during the procedure.

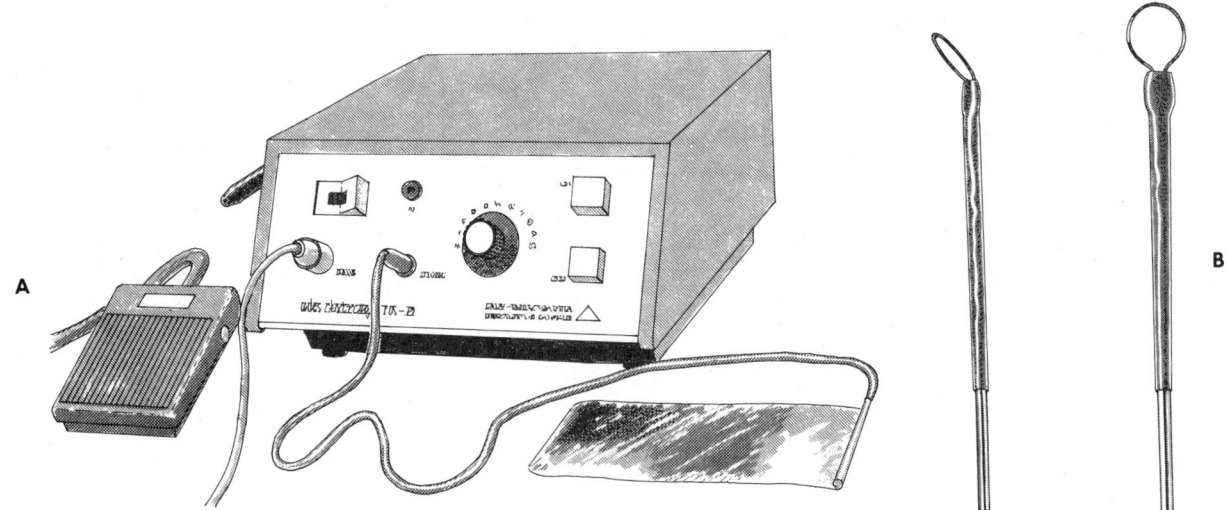

Fig. 9-22

10 ORAL SURGERY INSTRUMENTS

Pamela M. Peters

Oral maxillofacial surgery is defined by the American Board of Maxillofacial Surgery as "that part of dental practice which deals with the diagnosis, the surgical and adjunctive treatment of the diseases, injuries, and defects of the human jaws and associated structures." The accomplishment of these procedures requires special techniques and instruments.

Surgical instruments, with a few variations, are composed of the same parts as most other dental instruments. The nib or blade contains the cutting edge, the shank connects the handle and the blade, and the handle is held by the operator. The major addition to a number of surgical instruments is called the beak. The beak is a claw-shaped extension at the end of extraction forceps. Beaks, which contain a cutting edge, fit into the bifurcations of the teeth and, when various pressures are applied, prepare a tooth for removal.

Certain factors should be considered when selecting and using surgical instruments. The instrument must be made of a steel that can be sterilized frequently without rusting and that is soft enough to allow for the sharpening of cutting edges. The beaks and cutting edges must also be easy to keep clean. Finally, because of the design and weight of many of these instruments, a palm grasp is required.

Surgical instruments are available in many shapes and sizes. Each operator will have preferences. Familiarity with the basic design and function of each instrument will facilitate the dental team's ability to adapt to the instruments and overall procedures utilized by a specific dentist.

Scalpel handle and disposable blade (Fig. 10-1)

Physical characteristics
1. Available also as a single instrument, but more commonly as a handle with disposable blades.
2. Blades available in a variety of designs and identified by number.
3. Noncutting edge of the blade assumes an angle that allows it to fit and lock into the handle.

Use
To make an incision into the soft tissue of the oral cavity.

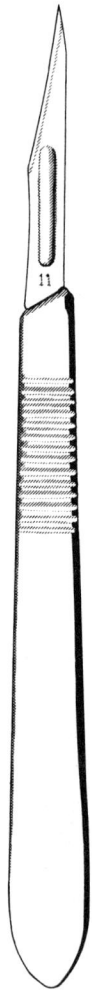

Fig. 10-1

ORAL SURGERY INSTRUMENTS

Periosteal elevator
(Fig. 10-2, A)

Physical characteristics
1. Single- or double-ended instrument.
2. Working end(s) parallel to the long axis of the handle.
3. Round or flat handle.
4. Working end(s) either wide and blunt or narrow and pointed.

Use
1. To separate and reflect the mucoperiosteum from the bone.
2. To retract the tissue to maintain access and view of the site.

Application (Fig. 10-2, B)
Retracts the tissue and exposes the surgical site.

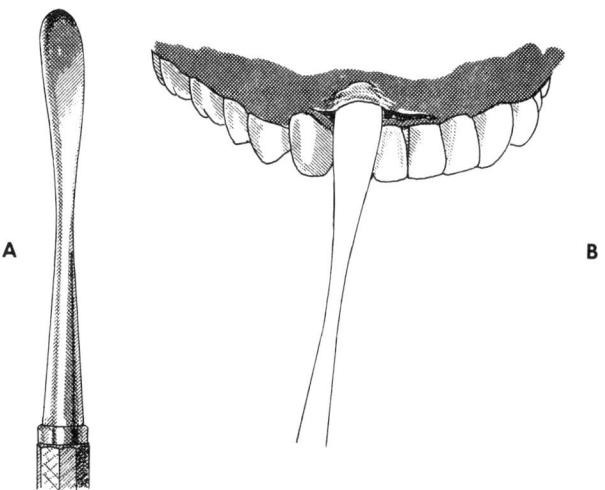

Fig. 10-2

Straight elevator
(Fig. 10-3, *A*)

Physical characteristics
1. Large, bulbous handle.
2. Working end resembles a sharp, narrow, elongated spoon.
3. Straight shank, parallel to the working end.

Use
1. To separate and loosen the tooth in its alveolus.
2. To remove large tooth fragments.

Application (Fig. 10-3, *B*)
Positioned between the tooth and its alveolus.

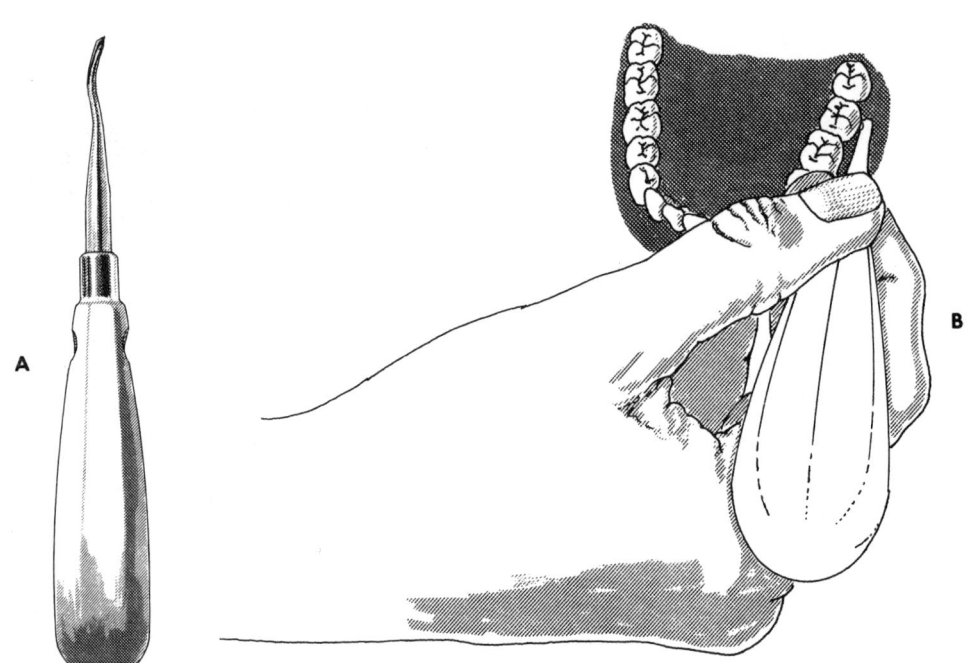

Fig. 10-3

ORAL SURGERY INSTRUMENTS

Apical elevator (root-tip pick) (Fig. 10-4, A)

Physical characteristics
1. Handle small in circumference.
2. Shanks either straight or contra-angled.
3. Working end small and delicate.
4. Similar but smaller than the straight elevator.

Use
To remove root tips.

Application (Fig. 10-4, B)
Removes a root tip from the socket.

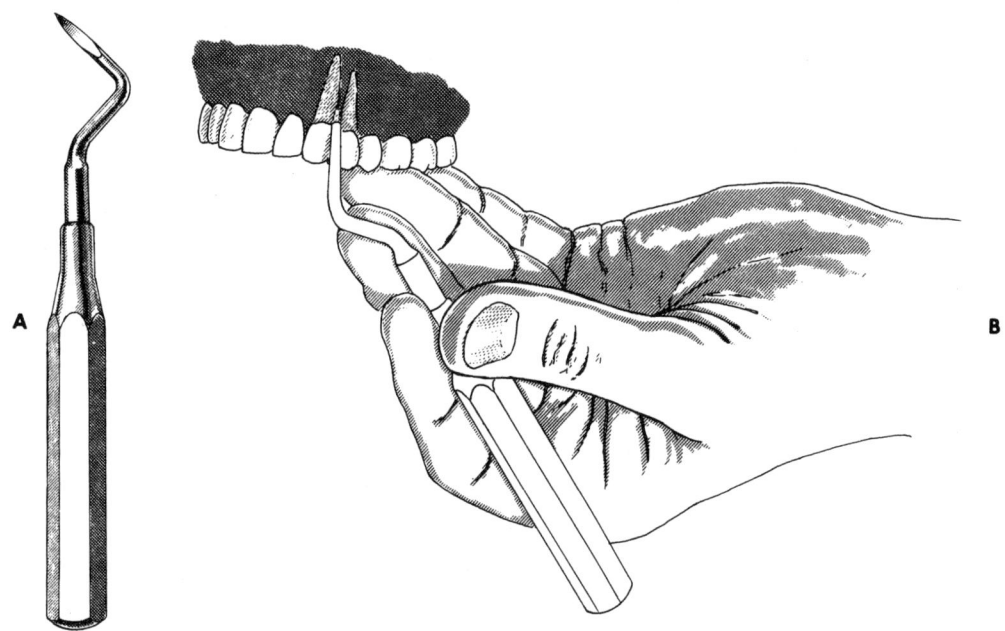

Fig. 10-4

Cryer elevator (Fig. 10-5)
T-bar elevator (Fig. 10-6)

Physical characteristics
1. Handles either large and bulbous or T shaped.
2. Working ends available in various designs.
3. Some produced in pairs, a right and a left.

Use
To remove root tips, especially those fractured during the extraction of multirooted teeth.

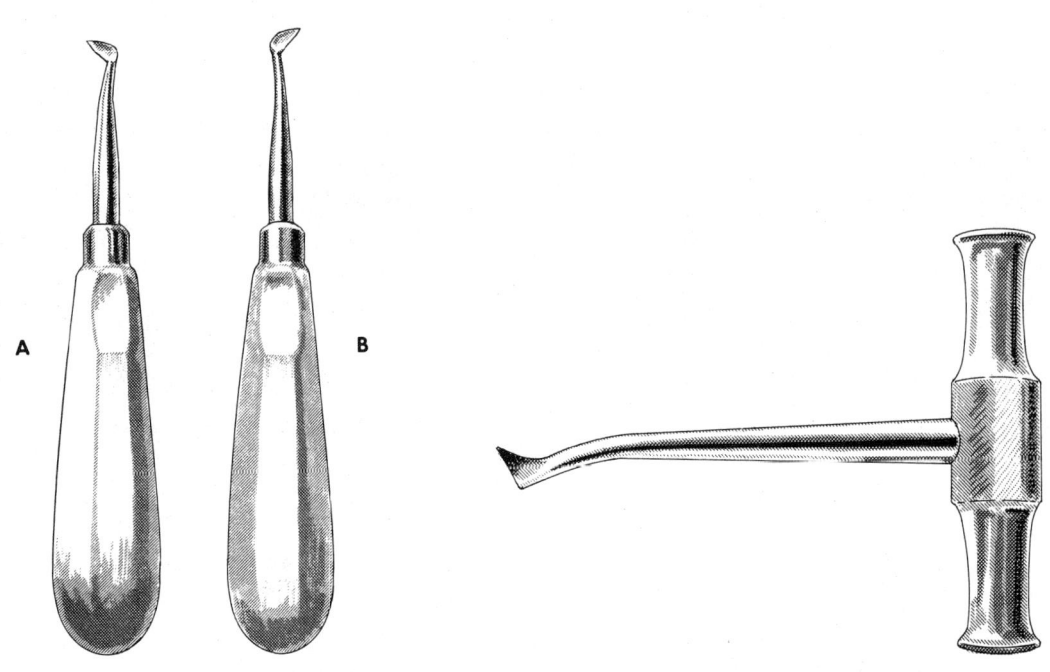

Fig. 10-5   Fig. 10-6

ORAL SURGERY INSTRUMENTS

Maxillary posterior extraction forceps (Fig. 10-7)
Universal maxillary forceps (Fig. 10-8)

Physical characteristics
1. Plierslike appearance.
2. Manufactured for use in both quadrants of the maxillary arch.
3. Beaks have smooth edges that allow them to fit around the bifurcated areas of all maxillary molar teeth.
4. Some made for use in only one quadrant of the maxillary arch; these have a point on the buccal beak that allows them to fit into the buccal bifurcation area.
5. An *R* next to the instrument number denotes use in the maxillary right quadrant, an *L* denotes use in the maxillary left quadrant.
6. Handles may be straight or have a curve at the end which allows the operator to utilize the instrument with greater pressure and stability.

Use
To extract maxillary posterior teeth from their alveoli.

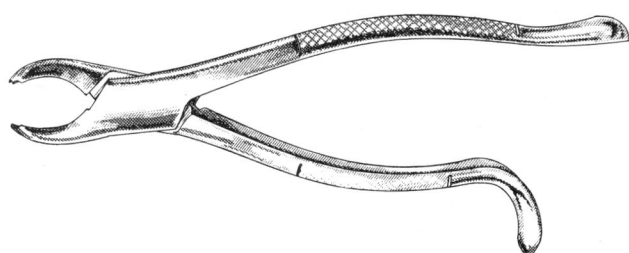

Fig. 10-7

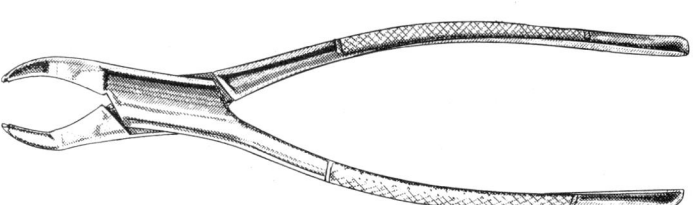

Fig. 10-8

Maxillary premolar extraction forceps
(Fig. 10-9)

Physical characteristics
1. Plierslike appearance.
2. Instruments with bayonet-shaped beaks are Universal.
3. Those designed for use on multirooted teeth available in pairs.

Use
To remove premolar teeth from their alveoli in the maxillary arch.

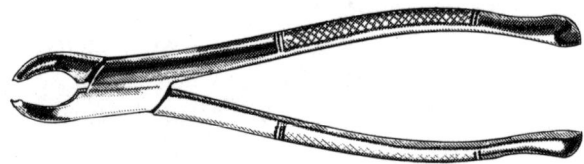

Fig. 10-9

Maxillary anterior extraction forceps
(Fig. 10-10)

Physical characteristics
1. Plierslike appearance.
2. Beaks straight and pointed.

Use
To extract any of the six maxillary anterior teeth.

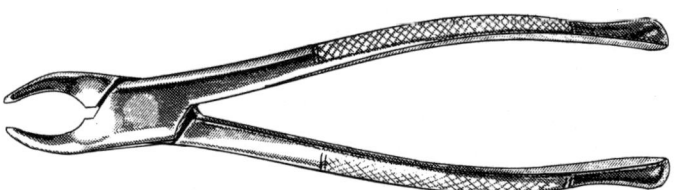

Fig. 10-10

Mandibular posterior extraction forceps
(Fig. 10-11, A)

Physical characteristics
1. Plierslike appearance.
2. Universal design and therefore functional in either quadrant of the arch.
3. Often referred to as a cowhorn forceps.

Use
To remove mandibular posterior teeth from their alveoli sockets.

Application
Fig. 10-11, B.

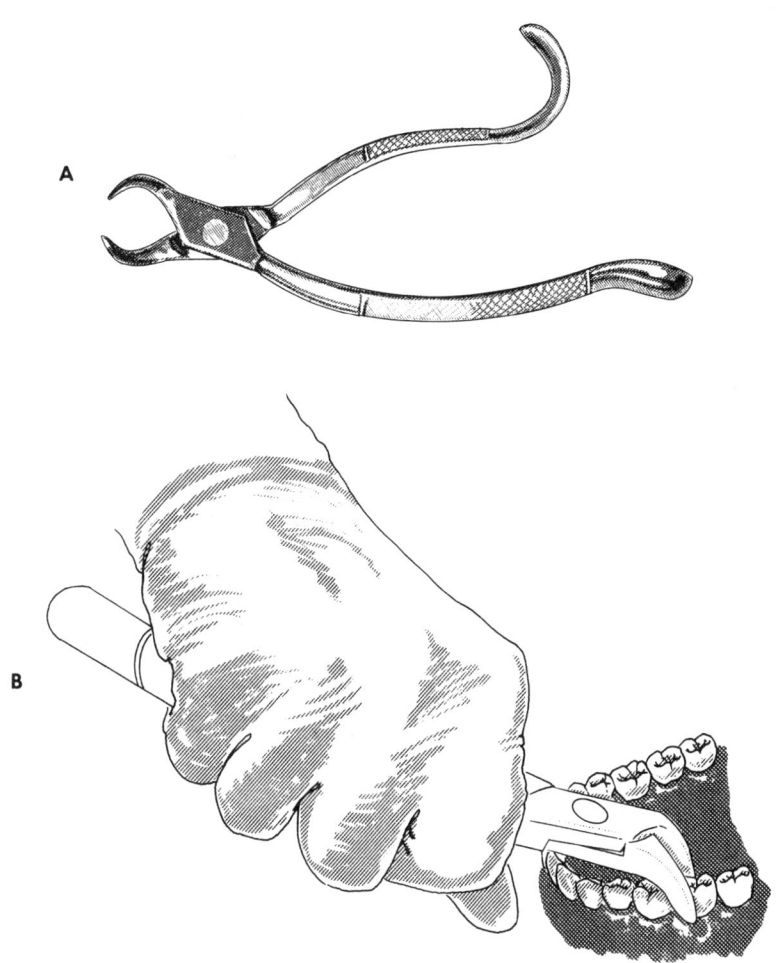

Fig. 10-11

ORAL SURGERY INSTRUMENTS

Mandibular incisor and premolar extraction forceps (Fig. 10-12)

Physical characteristics
1. Plierslike appearance.
2. Beaks designed to remove all mandibular teeth, but most often used on incisors and premolars.

Use
To extract mandibular incisor and premolar teeth.

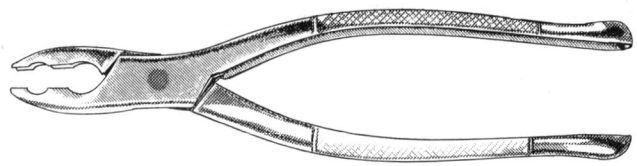

Fig. 10-12

Pedodontic extraction forceps (Fig. 10-13)

Physical characteristics
1. Design identical to forceps manufactured for use on permanent teeth.
2. Smaller in size than standard forceps.
3. Available in a variety of designs conducive to the extraction of teeth in specific areas of the oral cavity.

Use
To remove primary teeth from the oral cavity.

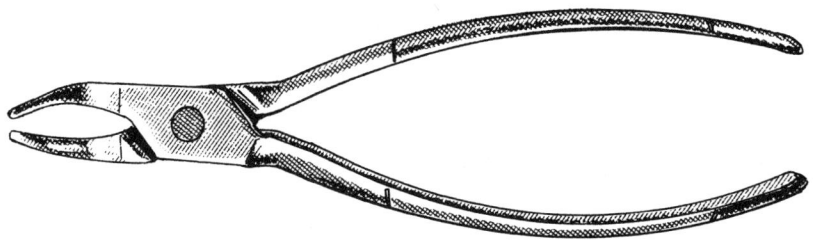

Fig. 10-13

ORAL SURGERY INSTRUMENTS

Curette (Fig. 10-14)

Physical characteristics
1. Long, thin handle.
2. Shank either straight or contra-angled.
3. Blade sharp and spoon shaped.
4. Available in a variety of sizes.

Use
1. Mainly to remove granulation or abnormal tissue from a tooth socket.
2. To sever the epithelial attachment of the gingiva prior to an extraction.

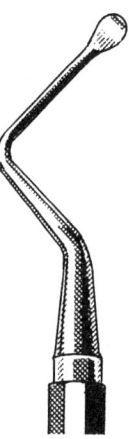

Fig. 10-14

Rongeur forceps
(Fig. 10-15, A and B)

Physical characteristics
1. Plierslike appearance.
2. Cutting surfaces of the blade on the end or on the sides.
3. Spring mechanism between the handles for stability.

Use
To trim or remove excess bone in a nipping fashion.

Application
Fig. 10-15, C.

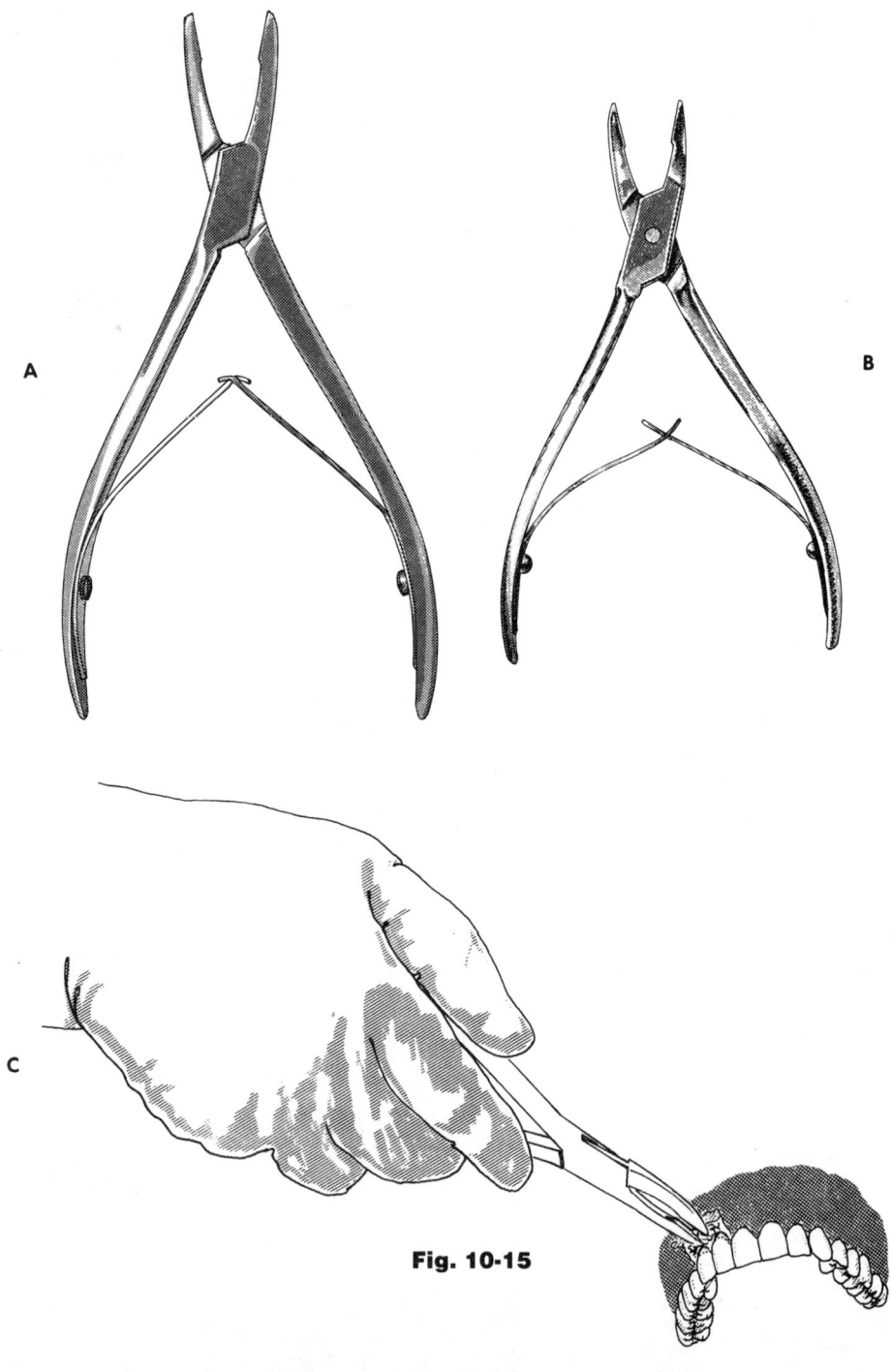

Fig. 10-15

ORAL SURGERY INSTRUMENTS

Bone file (Fig. 10-16)

Physical characteristics
1. Working end contains sharp serrations.
2. Available in single- and double-ended designs.
3. Variety of shapes and sizes.

Use

To remove or smooth rough edges of bone in a push-pull action.

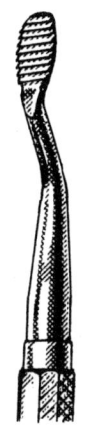

Fig. 10-16

Bone chisel (Fig. 10-17, *A*) **and surgical mallet** (Fig. 10-17, *B*)

Physical characteristics
Chisel
1. Length and width of the shaft vary.
2. Cutting end available in single-bevel and double-bevel designs.

Mallet
1. Hammer shaped.
2. Head available in lead or nylon.

Use
To trim or reshape bone to section teeth.

Application
Fig. 10-17, *C*.

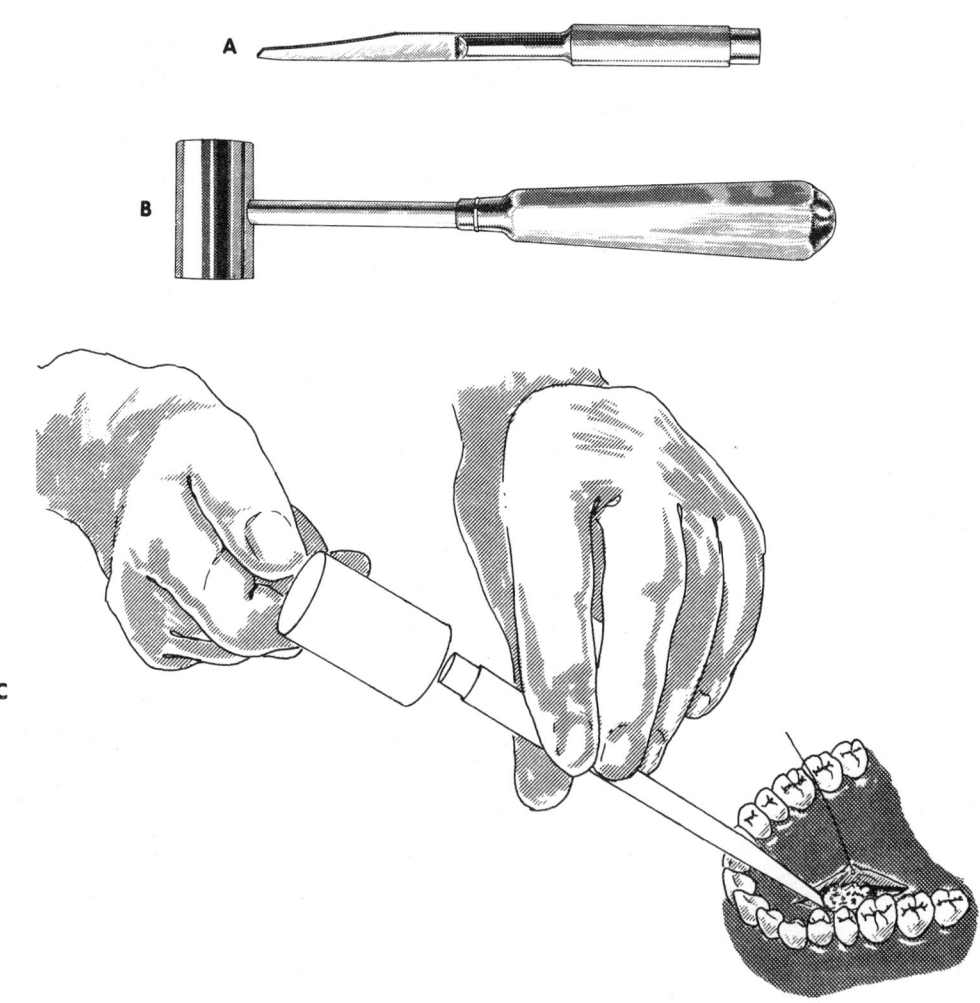

Fig. 10-17

ORAL SURGERY INSTRUMENTS

Surgical burs (Fig. 10-18)

Physical characteristics
1. Shanks longer than those of operative burs.
2. Used in both high- and low-speed handpieces.
3. Straight, crosscut fissure and large, round burs most commonly used.

Use

To remove bone and divide teeth for extraction purposes.

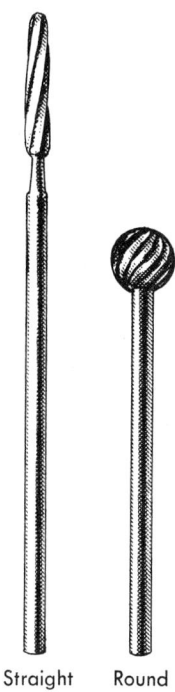

Straight Round

Fig. 10-18

Surgical scissors
(Fig. 10-19)

Physical characteristics
1. Cutting ends either sharp or blunt.
2. Handles and blades manufactured in straight and curved variations.
3. Blades available in smooth and serrated patterns.

Use
1. Scissors with sharp, delicate blades—mainly to trim soft tissue.
2. Scissors with less delicate blades—for such purposes as cutting suture material.

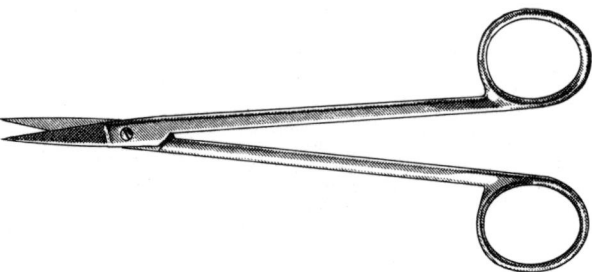

Fig. 10-19

ORAL SURGERY INSTRUMENTS

Hemostat (Fig. 10-20)

Physical characteristics
1. Scissorslike design.
2. Mechanical lock positioned between the handles.
3. Handles available in various lengths.
4. Serrated beaks either straight or curved.

Use
1. To grasp tissue, roots, or bone fragments.
2. Originally to clamp severed blood vessels.

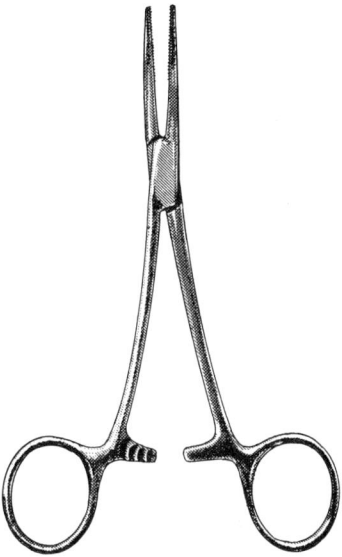

Fig. 10-20

Needle holder (Fig. 10-21)

Physical characteristics
1. Strongly resembles a hemostat.
2. Unlike hemostat's horizontal striations, inner surfaces of beak consist of a crisscross pattern.
3. Beaks contain a groove for grasping a needle.
4. Available in various lengths and shapes.

Use
To grasp and manipulate a needle during suturing procedures.

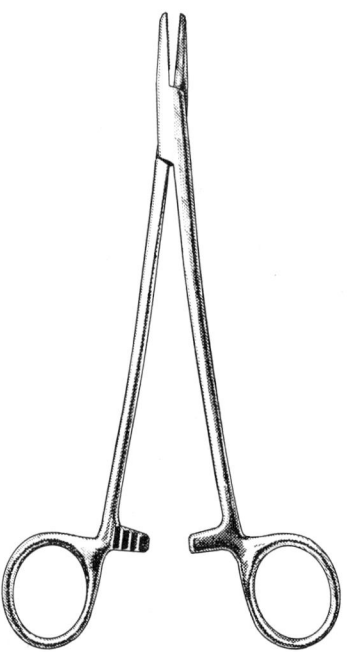

Fig. 10-21

11 INSTRUMENT SHARPENING

Christine P. Klausner
L. H. Klausner

Dental procedures can only be accomplished efficiently and effectively with sharp, accurate instruments. Repeated use and autoclaving of instruments leave the cutting edges dull and ineffective. A dull or irregular cutting surface:
1. Reduces the quality and precision required during instrumentation
2. Prolongs operating time
3. Necessitates the use of excessive force during instrumentation
4. Contributes to operator fatigue
5. Increases the risk of trauma to soft and hard tissues

Knowledge of the basic principles of instrument sharpening and development of the necessary skills to perform a sharpening technique are essential for a dental professional to practice effectively.

SHARPENING OBJECTIVE

The objective of instrument sharpening is to convert a flattened, dull surface into a sharp cutting edge while preserving the original blade shape.

The cutting edge of an instrument is created by the intersection of two surfaces of the blade forming a sharp angle. The cutting edge of a curette scaler, for example, is formed where the face of the blade meets the lateral surfaces (Fig. 11-1). On a sharp instrument, this intersection of two surfaces, which creates the cutting edge, forms a fine line. When an instrument becomes dull, the metal is worn away on the sharp edge, making it rounded or dulled. A rounded or flattened surface cuts only with excessive force, if at all.

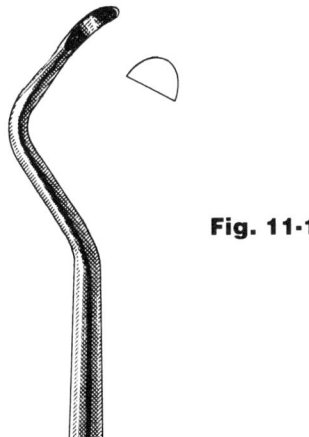

Fig. 11-1

SHARPNESS EVALUATION

There are two ways to evaluate instrument sharpness:
1. Cutting edges may be examined by looking at the edge under direct lighting. An instrument that is dull will reflect light, creating a glare, along the cutting edge when the instrument is slightly rotated (Fig. 11-2). This shiny reflection is caused by the flattened or rounded cutting surface. An instrument that is sharp will not reflect light along the edge. The use of a magnifying glass may assist in observing the instrument edge.
2. Tactile testing may also be used to determine instrument sharpness. The cutting edge is dragged across the thumbnail or the pad of a finger, using very light pressure. If the cutting edge "grabs" or "digs in" the nail or pad of the finger, the instrument is sharp. A dull instrument will slide easily over the nail or skin surface.

SHARPENING STONES

A sharpening stone is used to restore the sharp cutting edge on an instrument. Stones used for sharpening are made of abrasive particles, harder than the metal instrument, which grind the dull blade. Sharpening stones are made from:
1. Natural abrasives quarried from mineral deposits, such as India and Arkansas stones
2. Artificially produced stones, such as ruby stones, carborundum stones, Neivert whittlers, and diamond hones

The type of instrument to be sharpened determines which design, shape, and grit of sharpening stone will be used. The stones may be categorized by design and sharpening technique into three general types: mounted rotary stones, unmounted stones, and mechanical sharpeners.

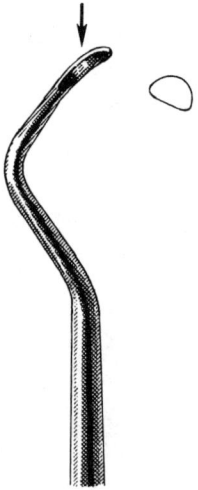

Fig. 11-2

INSTRUMENT SHARPENING

Mounted rotary stones
(Fig. 11-3)

1. Mandrel-mounted stones used with a motor-driven handpiece.
2. Cylindrical, conical, or disc-shaped. Cylindrical or conical stones suited for sharpening curved blades; disc-shaped stones facilitate sharpening of flattened blades, such as a spoon excavator or periodontal knife.
3. Various diameters available to fit different blade shapes.
4. Available in various grits.

This technique is not recommended for operators unskilled in using these stones. It is difficult to control the rotational speed of the stone and stabilize the instrument during the procedure. Improper technique may result in excessive removal of metal and altered blade shape.

Unmounted stones

1. Flat stones: rectangular with a flat or grooved surface (Fig. 11-4).
2. Hand stones: cylindrical or rectangular with rounded edges (Fig. 11-5).
3. Other types: Neivert whittler and diamond hone.
4. The sharpening technique requires manual manipulation of either the stone or the instrument while the other is held stationary.
5. A flat, mounted Arkansas stone is a general purpose stone that may be adapted for use on most instruments. A small, 1 × 2-inch (2.5 × 5-cm) stone is adequate for techniques requiring a stationary instrument and activated stone. A large, 1½ × 4-inch (3.8 × 10-cm) stone best for stationary stone techniques.
6. Cylindrical or conical stones limited to instruments with curved cutting edges.

A manual sharpening procedure using an unmounted stone is a good basic technique. It allows for more control of the stone to instrument angulation and less likelihood of removing too much metal or damaging instrument contour. It is, however, a more time-consuming process compared to the other techniques.

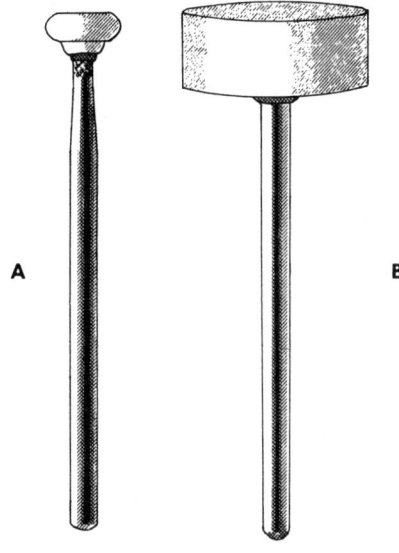

Fig. 11-3

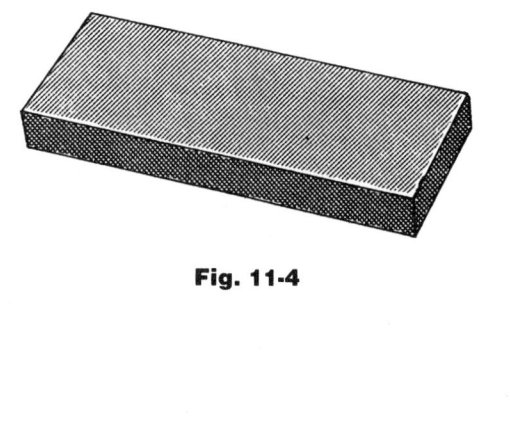

Fig. 11-4

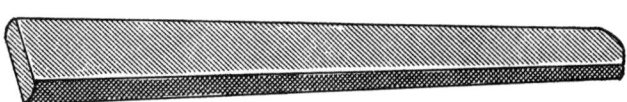

Fig. 11-5

Mechanical sharpeners

1. P_x honing machine (Fig. 11-6): provides rapid, reciprocating motion of a mounted stone in a horizontal direction. Various hone shapes and grits available to accommodate a variety of instruments.
2. Lathe-type mounted stones (Fig. 11-7): a large, circular Arkansas stone mounted on a motor-driven lathe. A guide may be provided in front of the stone to act as a rest and assist in maintaining the proper bevel of the instrument during sharpening.

Any mechanical sharpening is a time-saving technique, but requires much practice and maximum control. Instruments are easily oversharpened by grinding off too much metal and improperly contoured, reducing their usefulness.

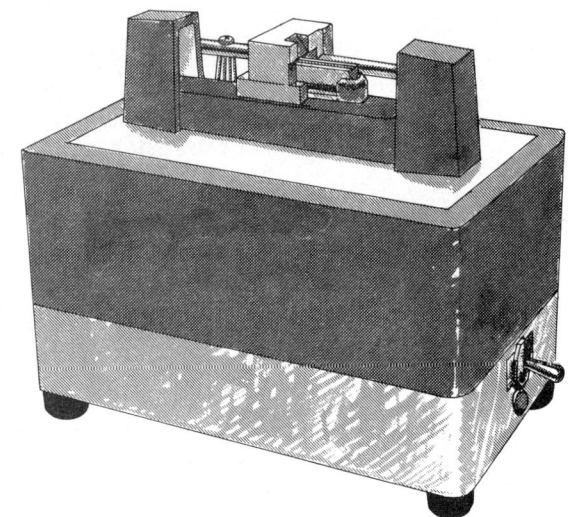

Fig. 11-6

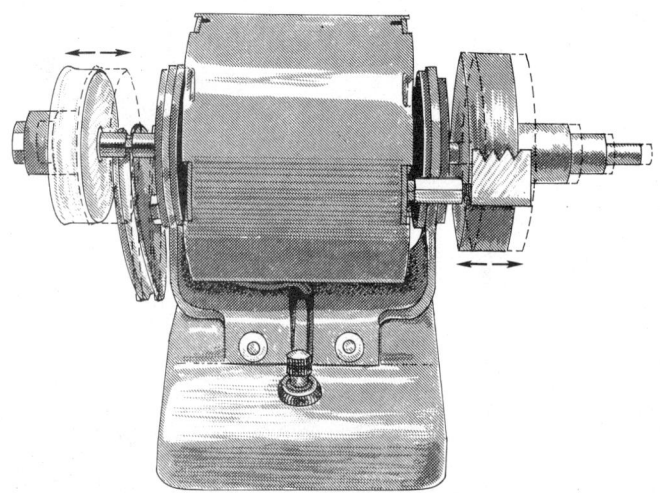

Fig. 11-7

INSTRUMENT SHARPENING

SHARPENING PRINCIPLES

1. For best results, sharpen instruments after sterilization because the sterilization procedure may dull a sharpened cutting edge.
2. Sharpen an instrument at the first indication of dullness. Excessively dull instruments are more difficult to sharpen and require removal of more metal to restore the cutting edge.
3. Select a stone and method of sharpening suitable for the instrument to be sharpened.
4. Develop a basic understanding of blade design and cutting edge angulation to prevent improper sharpening. Incorrect sharpening reduces instrument efficiency.
5. Keep the sharpening stone clean and oiled to maintain its cutting efficiency and to prevent overheating the instrument, which may result in loss of temper.
6. Use light pressure or a light stroke to remove as little metal as possible to obtain a sharp edge, and check frequently for sharpness.
7. Lightly hone (buff) the nonsharpened side of the instrument cutting edge with a few light strokes to remove any burs that may be created during sharpening.

SHARPENING HAND CUTTING INSTRUMENTS

A choice of a hand or mechanical sharpening technique may be used for such hand cutting instruments as hoes, chisels, hatchets, angle formers, and margin trimmers. A basic understanding of blade design is important before beginning any instrument sharpening (see previous chapters).

Hand sharpening technique (Fig. 11-8)

Hand sharpening is a more conservative approach to sharpening, requiring more time but less chance of instrument damage.

1. Lubricate an Arkansas stone with a thin layer of sterile, light machine oil.
2. Stabilize the stone on a flat surface.
3. Use a modified pen grasp to hold the instrument.
4. Maintain finger rests with the third and fourth fingers to assure stability during instrument activation.
5. Establish the correct bevel angulation on the stone. (The bevel is determined by the type of instrument sharpened.)
6. With a firm grasp, move the entire hand and arm together, directing the instrument in a back-and-forth motion, using about a 1-inch (2.5-cm) stroke length.
7. Wipe the instrument and check for sharpness. Repeat if necessary.
8. Hone the edge.

This technique is also useful for sharpening chisel and hoe scalers, which are similar in design to hand cutting instruments. Fig. 11-9 shows bevel placement for sharpening these two instruments; the arrow indicates the direction of the finishing stroke.

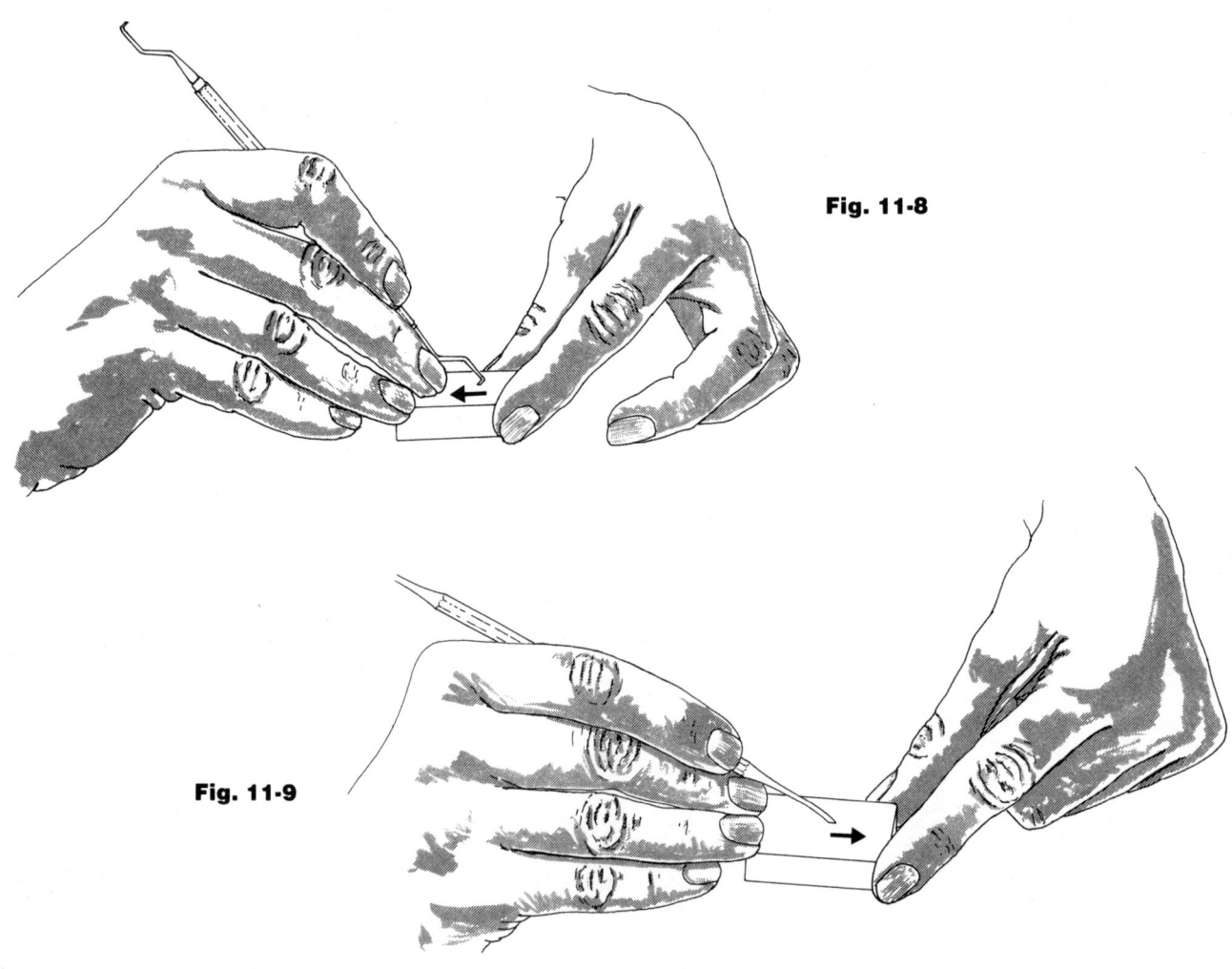

Fig. 11-8

Fig. 11-9

INSTRUMENT SHARPENING

Mechanical sharpening technique (Fig. 11-10)

Mechanical sharpening is a faster method, but care must be taken to avoid removing too much metal or altering instrument architecture.

1. Lubricate the grinding surface with an oil-soaked cotton roll.
2. Position the instrument so the entire bevel is contacting the grinding surface to maintain the original angulation. (Some mechanical sharpeners have a positioning guide.)
3. Using a firm, pen grasp, gently hold the instrument against the grinding edge for 1 to 2 seconds.
4. Check the instrument for sharpness and correct bevel.
5. Lightly hone the cutting edge to remove any burs that may have formed on the cutting edge.

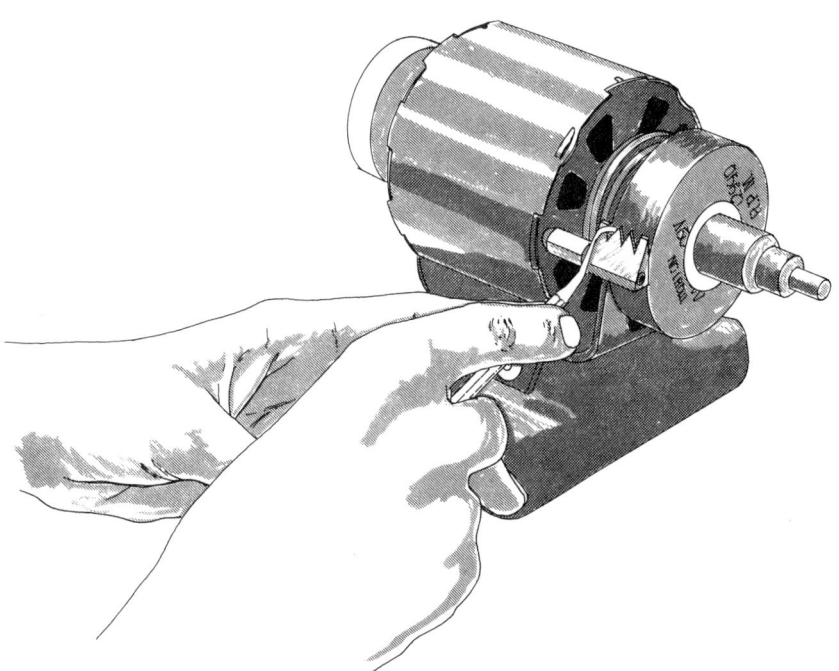

Fig. 11-10

SHARPENING CURETTES AND SICKLES

The blade design and importance of maintaining instrument contour indicate hand sharpening for curette and sickle scalers. These techniques are less likely to result in damage to the blade and help ensure a useful instrument life.

Moving stone and stationary instrument technique (Fig. 11-11)

1. Place a thin layer of sterile, light machine oil on an Arkansas stone.
2. Stabilize the instrument on the edge of a counter top with the fingers of one hand. The face of the scaler should be parallel to the floor, facing up.
3. Hold the stone with the length aligned in a vertical direction, using the fingers of the other hand.
4. Since the blade face is at a 90-degree angle to the stone, tilt the stone slightly away from the instrument, creating a 100- to 110-degree face-to-stone angle.
5. Working from the heel to the tip, begin short, up-and-down strokes, about ½ inch (1.3 cm) in length.
6. Finish with a down stroke.
7. Wipe the blade and check for sharpness. Repeat the sharpening if necessary.
8. Hone the edge.
9. Sharpen the opposite cutting edge.

The rounded configuration of the curette scaler requires additional sharpening after sharpening the lateral cutting edge. To sharpen the round tip:

10. Tilt the stone 135 degrees from the face. Using up-and-down strokes, gradually rotate the stone around the tip.
11. Repeated sharpening may alter the rounded contour of the curette base. Use short, brushlike strokes to remove angles that may develop on the base.

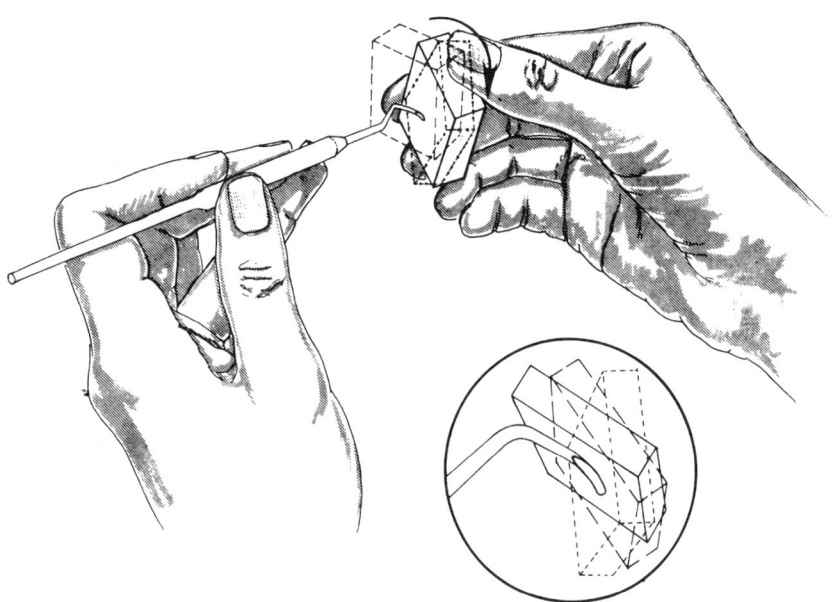

Fig. 11-11

INSTRUMENT SHARPENING

Moving instrument and stationary stone technique (Fig. 11-12)

1. Prepare an Arkansas stone with a thin layer of sterile, light machine oil.
2. Stabilize the stone on a flat surface.
3. Use a modified pen grasp to hold the instrument.
4. Maintain a finger rest with the third and fourth fingers.
5. Position the instrument blade on the stone. Maintain the blade face-to-stone angulation at 100 to 110 degrees.
6. Using moderate pressure, pull the instrument toward you, working from heel to tip. Rotate the instrument as the stroke progresses to the tip.
7. Wipe the blade and check for sharpness. Repeat the sharpening if necessary.
8. Sharpen the opposite cutting edge.
9. Hone the edges.

Use this procedure to sharpen outside cutting edges of instruments with angled shanks and both cutting edges of the straight sickle. Use the same procedure for sharpening inside cutting edges, only modify the instrument-to-stone placement. Place the cutting edge on the side of the stone, maintaining finger rests on the flat surface.

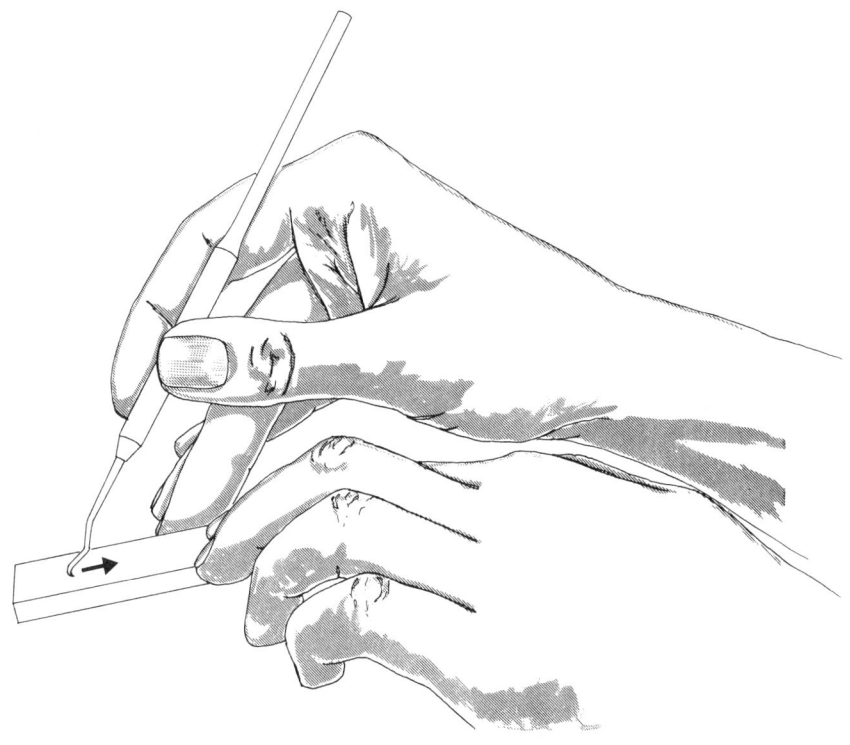

Fig. 11-12

CARE OF SHARPENING STONES

1. Lubricate the stone with sterile, light machine oil before sharpening. This helps prevent clogging of the surface of the stone with metal particles that reduce the abrasive action.
2. Wipe the stone with clean oil after use to remove metal particles and old oil accumulated during sharpening.
3. Clean the stone with ammonia, gasoline, or kerosene if it becomes blackened or clogged.
4. If the stone becomes glazed from repeated use and has lost its abrasive qualities, rub it over fine emery paper placed on a flat surface to resurface it.
5. Store stones in a covered container with a light coat of oil to prevent drying.
6. Use a sterile stone to sharpen sterile instruments that will be used on a patient. This prevents bacterial transfer. Autoclaving or hot oil techniques can be used to sterilize the stone.

12 INSTRUMENT STERILIZATION

Loretta M. Carter

A profession engaged in delivering health care must be concerned with infection. It is imperative that sterilization of dental instruments be a routine procedure in every dental office. Various methods of disinfection and sterilization can be employed to reduce the probability of infection and cross-contamination. It is mandatory that the dental team understand and properly use these methods.

INSTRUMENT PREPARATION

Cleaning dental instruments prior to sterilization or disinfection is essential and can be accomplished by either hand scrubbing or ultrasonic cleaning.

The ultrasonic cleaner (Fig. 12-1) provides the most effective method. Ultrasonic waves successfully vibrate small particles from the surfaces of the instruments.

Various solutions are available to be placed in the ultrasonic cleaner. These solutions are designed to remove gypsum products from impression trays and to remove cement from gold castings.

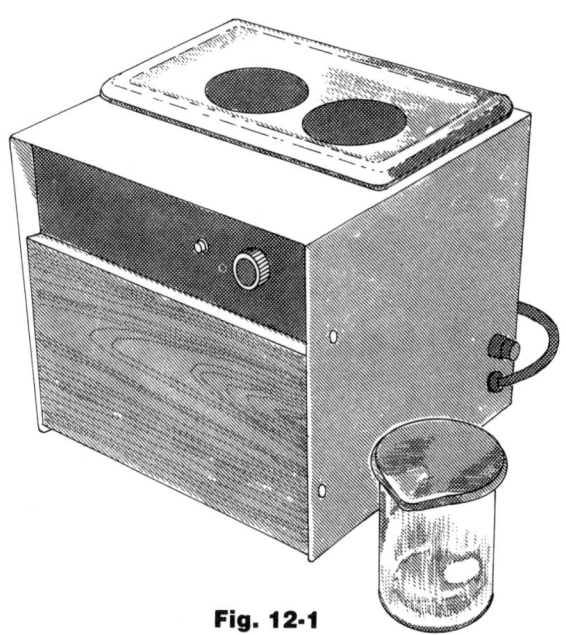

Fig. 12-1

STERILIZATION

Sterilization is the act of destroying all forms of life. The most accepted methods in dentistry and medicine for achieving *true* sterilization are extended periods of high heat and steam heat.

Steam heat sterilization

A steam heat sterilizer is available in various designs and sizes, depending on the size and number of instruments to be processed daily (Fig. 12-2). Steam is created in the sterilizing chamber by heating the water to its boiling point of 212° F (100° C). The steam (under pressure) created inside the sterilizing chamber must reach a temperature of 250° F (121° C) for a minimum of 15 minutes to successfully destroy heat-resistant bacterial forms.

It is necessary to protect the delicate cutting edges and hinged points of dental instruments because of the corrosive effect of steam on metal. Two methods available to accomplish this are an emulsifying bath and an ammonia-base bath spray. The emulsifying bath (Fig. 12-3, *A*) is a milk-oil solution that will not homogenize. The oil remains on the surface of the instrument, lubricating and protecting the instrument from corrosion. The ammonia-base spray (Fig. 12-3, *B*) creates an atmospheric change within the chamber of the autoclave with a similar result as the emulsifying bath.

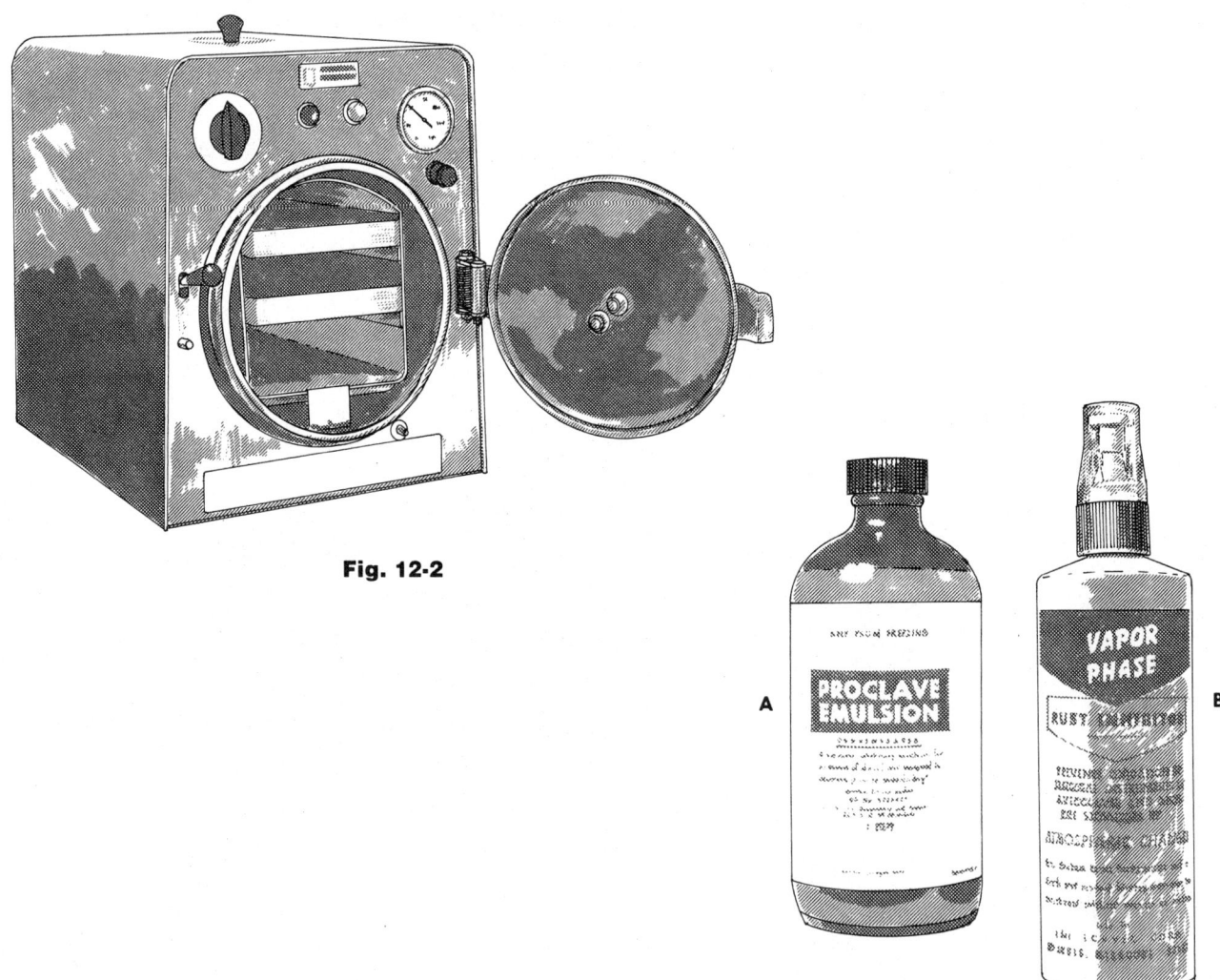

Fig. 12-2

Fig. 12-3

INSTRUMENT STERILIZATION

Dry-heat sterilization Dry-heat sterilization has become a preferred method of sterilization (Fig. 12-4). The process is efficient, effective, and relatively inexpensive. Dental instuments may be placed inside or on heat-resistant trays and placed directly into the "oven" for processing. The preparatory stage used for autoclaving dental instruments is not necessary for dry-heat sterilization because steam is not employed with this method. The temperature for a dry-heat sterilizer is lower and therefore must be maintained for a longer period to be effective.

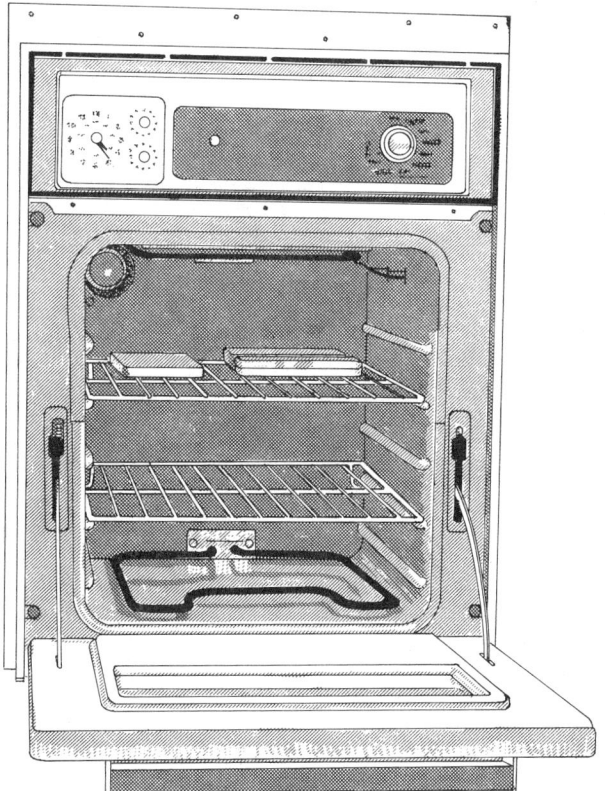

Fig. 12-4

Chemical sterilization   The chemical sterilizer is a relatively new method for sterilization of dental instruments (Fig. 12-5). The concept is the same as steam under pressure, except a chemical solution rather than water is employed. In contrast to the autoclave, instruments must be completely dried for the chemical sterilizer, and no spray or emulsifying agent is necessary. The combination of water and chemical vapor would have a corrosive effect on the instrument surface.

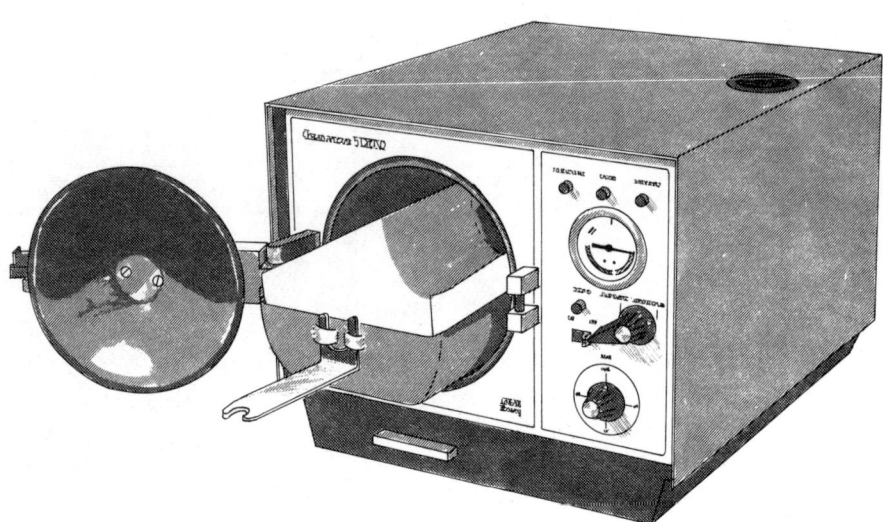

Fig. 12-5

INSTRUMENT STERILIZATION

Bead sterilization   The bead sterilizer (Fig. 12-6) was developed for endodontic instruments. It consists of a small pot of glass beads or salt maintained at a temperature of 450° F (250° C). This is an accepted method for resterilization of reamers, files, and broaches. The instruments should be placed into the beads or salt for approximately 15 to 20 seconds.

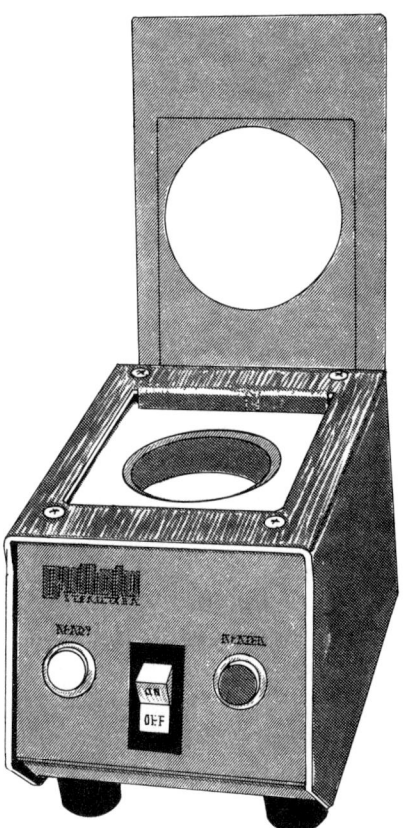

Fig. 12-6

DISINFECTION Disinfection only inhibits the growth of disease-causing microorganisms and is not nearly as effective as sterilization. Only dental instruments that cannot withstand the high temperature of heat sterilization should be placed in a disinfectant solution.

Some of the chemicals available for use as disinfectants are benzalkonium chloride, hexachlorophene, and rubbing alcohol. All of these chemicals should be used as directed. Stronger concentrations of a solution will not be *more* effective.

A more popular term for chemical disinfection is "cold sterilization." The instruments are placed in an open disinfectant bath (Fig. 12-7) for the required length of time.

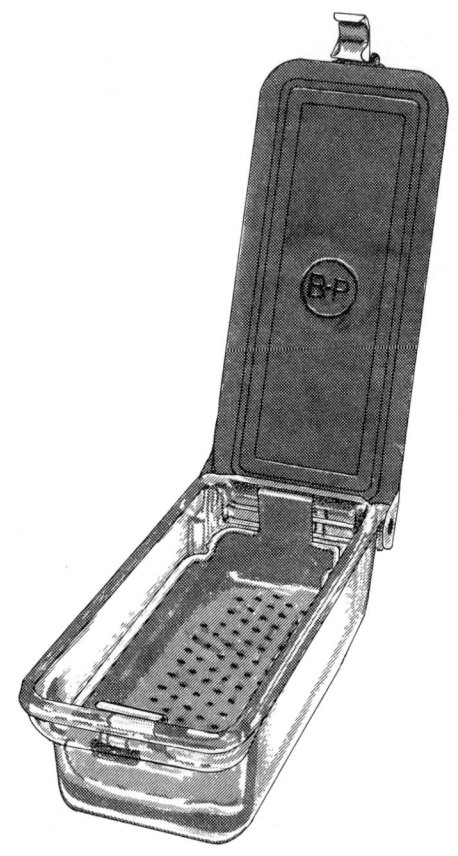

Fig. 12-7

INSTRUMENT STERILIZATION

Hot oil sterilizer
(Fig. 12-8)

Dental handpieces, as well as dental hand instruments, must be lubricated and cleaned. This is not considered a sterilization method, but rather a disinfecting and lubricating one. Dental handpieces are immersed into a bath of oil that has been heated to 320° F (178° C) for approximately 15 to 20 minutes.

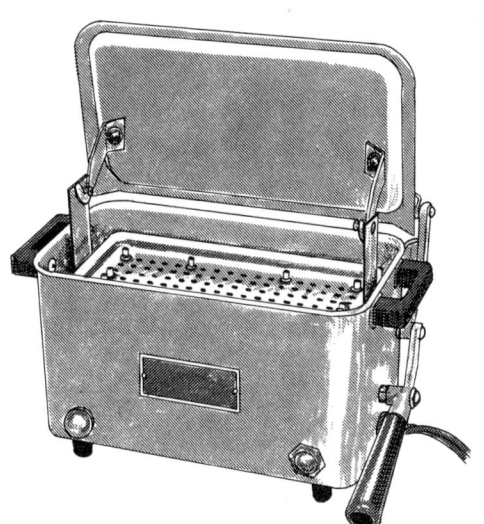

Fig. 12-8

BIBLIOGRAPHY

1. Advanced speeds in operative dentistry, 1967, Bureau of Naval Personnel.
2. Bell, B. H., and Grainger, D. A.: Basic operative dentistry procedures, ed. 2, Philadelphia, 1971, Lea & Febiger.
3. Bence, R.: Handbook of clinical endodontics, St. Louis, 1976, The C. V. Mosby Co.
4. Black, G. V.: Operative dentistry, vol. 2, Chicago, 1908, Medico-Dental Publishing Co.
5. Black, G. V.: A work on operative dentistry in two volumes, ed. 6, Chicago, 1924, Medico-Dental Publishing Co.
6. British Medical Association: Lecture memoranda: the dental art in ancient times, London, 1914, Burroughs & Welcome Co.
7. Carranza, F. F.: Glickman's clinical periodontology, ed. 5, Philadelphia, 1979, W. B. Saunders Co.
8. A century of service to dentistry, Philadelphia, 1944, S. S. White Dental Manufacturing Co.
9. Charbeneau, G. T., and others: Principles and practice of operative dentistry, ed. 3, Philadelphia, 1975, Lea & Febiger.
10. Chasteen, J. E.: Essentials of clinical dental assisting, St. Louis, 1975, The C. V. Mosby Co.
11. Coleman, A. I.: History of dentistry, Syllabus, 1976, University of Southern California.
12. Costich, E. R., and White, R. P.: Fundamentals of oral surgery, Philadelphia, 1971, W. B. Saunders Co.
13. Dunn, A., Booth, D. F., and Clancy, M.: Pharmacology, pain control, sterile technique, oral surgery, Baltimore, 1975, The Williams & Wilkins Co.
14. Gilmore, H. W., and others: Operative dentistry, ed. 3, St. Louis, 1977, The C. V. Mosby Co.
15. Glickman, I.: Clinical periodontology, ed. 4, Philadelphia, 1972, W. B. Saunders Co.
16. Green, E., and Seyer, P. C.: Sharpening curettes and sickle scalers, San Francisco, 1972, Praxis Publishing Co.
17. Horty, F. J., and Roberts, D. H.: Restorative procedures for the practicing dentist, Bristol, 1974, John Wright & Sons, Ltd.
18. Ingle, J. I., and Beveridge, E. E.: Endodontics, ed. 2, Philadelphia, 1976, Lea & Febiger.
19. Ingraham, R., and Koser, J. R.: An atlas of gold foil and rubber dam procedures, Buena Park, Calif., 1961, Uni-Tro College Press.
20. Johnson & Lund: Catalogue of dentists' materials, Philadelphia, 1871.
21. Johnson & Lund: Purchaser's guide, Philadelphia, 1876.
22. Pawlak, E. A., and Hoag, P. M.: Essentials of periodontics, ed. 2, St. Louis, 1980, The C. V. Mosby Co.
23. Pickard, H. M.: A manual of operative dentistry, London, 1961, Oxford University Press.
24. Richardson, R. E., and Barton, R. E.: The dental assistant, ed. 5, New York, 1978, McGraw-Hill Book Co.
25. Robinson, J. B.: The foundations of professional dentistry, Baltimore, 1940, Waverly Press.
26. Ross, J. R., Kimmelman, J. R., and Miller, P. D.: Determining the need for periodontal surgery. III, Surgical instruments: their use and care, J. Acad. Gen. Dent., 1975.
27. Schwarzrock, S. P., and Jensen, J. R.: Effective dental assisting, ed. 5, Dubuque, Iowa, 1978, William C. Brown Co.
28. SSW instrument catalog, 1972, Division of Pennwalt Corporation.
29. Sturdevant, C. M., Barton, R. E., and Brauer, J. C.: The art and science of operative dentistry, New York, 1968, McGraw-Hill Book Co.
30. Torres, H. O., and Ehrlich, A.: Modern dental assisting, Philadelphia, 1976, W. B. Saunders Co.
31. Ward, H., and Simring, M.: Manual of clinical periodontics, ed. 2, St. Louis, 1978, The C. V. Mosby Co.
32. Weine, F. S.: Endodontic therapy, ed. 2, St. Louis, 1976, The C. V. Mosby Co.
33. Wilkens, E. M.: Clinical practice of the dental hygienist, ed. 4, Philadelphia, 1976, Lea & Febiger.

INDEX

INDEX

A

Absorbent wafer, 21
Adjustable articulator, 10
Agents, polishing, 135
Alcohol lamp, 58
Aluminum oxide abrasive, 47
Amalgam carrier, 54-55
   micro-sized retro, 92
Amalgam condensing instruments, 52-57
Amalgam plugger, serrated, 97
American Board of Maxillofacial Surgery, 147
Angle, prophylaxis, 131
Angulated bracket-removing pliers, 102
Anterior extraction forceps, maxillary, 154
Anterior-band–removing pliers, 108
Apical elevator, 151
Arch marker, 106
Arch-adjusting pliers, Tweed, 93
Arch-forming pliers, 113
Aristotle and dental history, 1
Articulation paper pliers, 6
Articulator, 10
Automatic band driver, 100
Automatic hand condenser, 61

B

"B" burnisher, 100
Bachus towel clamp, 12
Band biter, 95
Band burnisher, 100
Band driver, automatic, 100
Band pusher, Mershon, 95
Band seater, nylon molar, 95
Band-contouring pliers, 106
Band-removing pliers, posterior, 105
Bands, 107
Band-seating file, 100
Band-slitting and -removing pliers, 102
Bases, direct-bond, 102
Basic enamel hatchet, 34-35
Bead sterilization, 178
Bevel of chisels, 29
Biangle chisels, 32
Biangle shank, 28
Biangle-angle chisels, 34
Bird-beak, 94
Biter, band, 95
Black, G.V., and dental history, 3
Blade of instrument, 26
   disposable, and scalpel handle, 148
Bone chisel, 160
Bone files, 145, 159
Bracket-removing pliers, angulated, 102

Brackets, direct-bond, 102
Bristle brushes, 132
Broach, 83
Brushes, bristle, 132
Bur shapes, 44
Burnisher, 66
   band, 100
Burs, 43-45
   micro-sized, 91
   surgical, 91, 161

C

Canal, root
   obturation instruments, 86-90
   preparation of, contra-angles for, 84-85
Carrier
   amalgam, 54-55
      micro-sized retro, 92
   cohesive gold, 59
Celsus, Cornelius, and dental history, 1
Chemical sterilization, 178
Chevalier and dental history, 2
Chisel(s), 29-34
   bone, 160
   hard-tissue surgical, 143
Chisel scaler, 124
Circular rubber dam frame, 14
Clamp(s)
   Bachus towel, 12
   rubber dam, 15, 77
Clasp adjusting pliers, 99
Cleaner, ultrasonic, 175
Cleaning instruments, 131-145
"Cold sterilization," 180
Collar and crown scissors, 73
Cohesive gold carrier, 59
Cohesive gold hand condenser, 60
Cohesive gold instruments, 58-67
Condenser(s)
   hand
      automatic, 61
      cohesive gold, 60
      mechanical, 54, 62
Condenser points, 61
Condensing instruments, amalgam, 52-57
Cones, silver, 86
Contra-angle(s)
   micro–, 91
   for root canal preparation, 84-85
Contra-angle handpieces, 41
Coon ligature-tying pliers, 104
Cotton pliers, 6

Cotton roll holders, 21
Cotton rolls, 20
Cowhorn forceps, 155
Cowhorn style explorer, 4
Crown and collar scissors, 73
Cryer elevator, 152
Cup, rubber polishing, 132
Curettes, 128-129, 157
   sharpening, 172-174
   surgical, 141
Cutter(s)
   ligature-wire, 110
   with parallel-action pliers, 118
Cutting instruments, hand, 26-28
Cylindrical plastic endodontic instruments, 72

D

D-11 endodontic spreaders, 87
Dam, rubber, 13, 19, 79
   clamps, 15, 77
   forceps, 17, 78
   frame, 14, 76
   gauze mask, 18
   punch, 16, 78
Dappen dish, 7
Dental floss and tape, 134
Diamond hone, 167
Diamond points, 46
Direct-bond brackets and bases, 102
Director, ligature, 101
Discs, 48
Disinfection, 180-181
Disposable blade and scalpel handle, 148
Distal-end–cutting pliers and holder, 114
Drill, Gates Glidden, 84
Driver, automatic band, 100
Dry-heat sterilization, 177

E

Ejector, saliva, 22-23
Ejector system, vacuum, 124-125
Elastic pliers, separating, 98
Electrosurgical instruments, 146
Elevator
   apical, 151
   Cryer, 152
   periosteal, 139, 149
   straight, 150
   T-bar, 152
Enamel hatchet, basic, 34-35
Endodontic explorer, 4
Endodontic instruments, 68-92
Engine-driven reamer, 84

Evacuator, high-volume, 24-25
Examination instruments, periodontal, 119-121
Excavator, spoon, 38
   long-shank, 69
Explorer, 4, 119
   endodontic, 71
Extraction forceps
   mandibular posterior, 155
   maxillary
     anterior, 154
     posterior, 153
     premolar, 154
   pedodontic, 156
   premolar, 156

F

Face-bow–adjusting pliers, 111
Fauchard, Pierre, and dental history, 2
File(s)
   band-seating, 100
   bone, 145, 159
   gold, 64
   Hedstrom, 82
   K-type, 82
   root canal, 81
File scaler, 126-127
Filler, paste, Lentulo-type, 90
Filling instruments, retrograde, 91
Filling materials, 86
Fillings, paste, 86
Finger spreader and plugger, 89
Finishing burs, plug, 45
Flagg, J. Foster, and dental history, 2
Flame-shaped finishing burs, 45
Flat stones, 167
Floss, dental, 134
Forceps, 6
   cowhorn, 155
   mandibular extraction
     incisor and premolar, 156
     posterior, 155
   maxillary
     extraction
       anterior, 154
       posterior, 153
       premolar, 154
       universal, 153
   pedodontic extraction, 156
   rongeur, 158
   rubber dam, 17, 78
Frame, rubber dam, 14, 76
Friction-grip bur, 43
Friction-grip head contra-angle handpieces, 41

INDEX

Friction-grip head mandrels, screw, 50

G

Galen and dental history, 1
Gates Glidden drill, 84
Gingival margin trimmers, 36-37
Giromatic contra-angle, 85
Gold, cohesive
    carrier, 59
    hand condenser, 60
    instruments, 58-67
Gold file, 64
Gold knife, 65
Green stones, 47
Gutta-percha, 86

H

Hand condenser
    automatic, 61
    cohesive gold, 60
Hand cutting instruments, 26-38
    sharpening, 169-171
Hand mallet, 63
Hand mirrors, 5
Hand sharpening technique, 170
Hand stones, 167
Handle of instrument, 26
    scalpel, and disposable blade, 148
Handpieces, 40-42
Hard-tissue surgical instruments, 143-145
Hatchets, 34-38
Head of bur, 43
Heat sterilization
    dry, 177
    steam, 176
Hedstrom files, 82
Hemostat, 163
High-speed handpieces, 42
High-volume evacuator, 24-25
History of dental instruments, 1-3
Hoe scaler, 125
Hoes, 33
    hard-tissue surgical, 143
Holder(s)
    cotton roll, 21
    distal-end–cutting, 114
Hone, diamond, 167
Hot oil sterilizer, 181
Howe utility pliers, 103
HVE; *see* High-volume evacuator

I

Impression trays, orthodontic, 109

Incisor forceps, mandibular, 156
Intracanal instruments, 82
Intraoral photography mirrors, 5
Irrigation syringe, endodontic, 75
Isolation, instruments for, 13-25
Ivory porte polisher, 133
Ivory retainers, 56
Ivory rubber dam clamps, 77

J

Jacquette sickle scaler, 122, 123

K

Knife(ves)
    gold, 63
    periodontal, 138
K-type file, 82

L

Lamp, alcohol, 58
Latch bur, 43
Latch head contra-angle handpieces, 41
Latch head mandrel
    pinhead screw, 50
    screw, 50
    snap, 50
Latch head prophylaxis angle, 131
Lentulo-type paste filler, 90
Lewis, John, and dental history, 2
Ligature director, 101
Ligature pliers, 117
Ligatures, 18
Ligature-tying pliers, Coon, 104
Ligature-wire cutters, 110
Light-wire pliers, 112
Locking pliers, endodontic, 70
Long-shank spoon excavator, 69
Loop-forming pliers, Tweed, 116
Low-speed handpieces, 40-41
Luer-Lok syringe, 75
Luks pluggers, 88

M

Mallet
    hand, 63
    surgical, 160
Mandibular forceps
    incisor, 156
    posterior extraction, 155
Mandrels, 50
Manual polishing instruments, 133-135
Margin trimmers, gingival, 36-37
Marker

Marker—cont'd
  arch, 106
  periodontal pocket, 136-137
Mask, gauze, rubber dam, 18
Mathieu style pliers, 117
Matrices, 57
Matrix retainers, 56
Maxillary forceps
  extraction
    anterior, 154
    posterior, 153
    premolar, 154
  universal, 153
MCE-1 plastic endodontic instrument, 72
Mechanical condensers, 54, 62
Mechanical polishing instruments, 131-132
Mechanical separator, 67
Mechanical sharpeners, 168
Mechanical sharpening technique, 171
Mershon band pusher, 95
Micro–contra-angle, 91
Micro-sized burs, 91
Micro-sized retro amalgam carrier and pluggers, 92
Miller points, 52, 53
Mirrors, 5, 119
Mixing slabs and pads, 8
Molar band seater, nylon, 95
Molt mouth prop, 11
Monangle chisels, 30
Monangle shank, 28
Morrison and dental history, 2
Mounted rotary stones, 167
Mouth props, 11
Moving instrument and stationary stone technique, 173
Moving stone and stationary instrument technique, 172
Mynol porte polisher, 133

N

Needle holder, 164
Neivert whittler, 167
Nib of instrument, 26
No. 3 endodontic spreader, 87
No. 11 scalpels, 142
No. 12 scalpels, 142
No. 12B scalpels, 142
No. 15 scalpels, 142
Nygard-Ostby rubber dam frame, 76
Nylon molar band seater, 95

O

Obturation instruments, root canal, 86-90

Oil, hot, sterilizer, 181
Omega pliers, 116
Openers, orifice, 83
Operative Dentistry, 3
Oral surgery instruments, 147-164
Orangewood stick, 134
Orifice openers, 83
Orthodontic instruments, 93-118

P

Paddle-shaped plastic endodontic instruments, 72
Pads, mixing, 8
Paper, articulation, pliers, 6
Parallel-action pliers with cutter, 118
Paste filler, Lentulo-type, 90
Paste fillings, 86
Paul of Aegina and dental history, 2
Pear-shaped finishing burs, 45
Pedodontic extraction forceps, 156
Peeso reamer, 84
Periapical surgery instruments, endodontic, 91
Periodontal instruments, 119-146
Periosteal elevator, 139, 149
Pfingst racer contra-angle, 85
Photography, intraoral, mirrors for, 5
Pick, root-tip, 151
Plain line articulator, 10
Plastic endodontic instruments, 72
Pliers
  angulated bracket-removing, 102
  anterior-band–removing, 108
  arch-forming, 113
  band-contouring, 106
  band-slitting and -removing, 102
  clasp adjusting, 99
  Coon ligature-tying, 104
  cotton, 6
  distal-end–cutting, 114
  endodontic locking, 70
  face-bow–adjusting, 111
  Howe utility, 103
  ligature, 117
  light-wire, 112
  parallel-action with cutter, 118
  posterior band-removing, 105
  separating elastic, 98
  silver point, 86
  triple-beaked, 99
  Tweed arch-adjusting, 93
  Tweed loop-forming, 116
  Weingart utility, 115
Plug finishing burs, 45
Plugger(s)

INDEX

Plugger(s)—cont'd
  endodontic, 88
  finger, 89
  micro-sized retro amalgam, 92
  serrated amalgam, 97
Pocket marker, periodontal, 136-137
Point pliers, silver, 86
Points
  condenser, 61
  diamond, 46
Polishing agents, 135
Polishing cup, rubber, 132
Polishing instruments, 131-145
Polishing strips, 135
Porte polisher, 133
Posterior band-removing pliers, 105
Posterior extraction forceps
  mandibular, 155
  maxillary, 153
Premolar extraction forceps, 156
  maxillary, 154
Probe, periodontal, 120-121
Prophylaxis angle, 131
Props, mouth, 11
Punch, rubber dam, 16, 78
Pusher, Mershon band, 95

R

Racer Pfingst contra-angle, 85
Reamer, 82
  engine-driven, 84
  Peeso, 84
10:1 reduction contra-angle, 84
Retainers, matrix, 56
Retro amalgam carrier and pluggers, micro-sized, 92
Retrograde filling instruments, 91
Reverse bevel chisel, 29
Rhazes and dental history, 2
Right angle explorer, 4
Roll(s), cotton, 20
  holders, 21
Rongeur forceps, 158
Rongeurs, 144
Root canal files, 81
Root canal obturation instruments, 86-90
Root-tip pick, 151
Rotary instruments, 39-50, 84
Rotary stones, mounted, 167
Rotating instruments, 145-146
2-4-6 round finishing bur, 45
Rubber dam, 13, 19, 79
  clamps, 15, 77
  forceps, 17, 78

Rubber dam—cont'd
  frame, 14, 76
  gauze mask, 18
  punch, 16, 78
Rubber mouth prop, 11
Rubber polishing cup, 132
Ruler, endodontic, 74

S

Saliva ejector, 22-23
Sargent pliers, 118
Scaling instruments, 122-130
Scalpel handle and disposable blade, 148
Scalpels, 142
Scissors
  collar and crown, 73
  straight, 19
  surgical, 140, 162
Screw head mandrels, 50
Screw-type head prophylaxis angle, 131
Seater, nylon molar band, 95
Separating elastic pliers, 98
Separator, mechanical, 67
Serrated amalgam plugger, 97
Shaft
  of bur, 43
  of instrument, 26
Shank
  of bur, 43
  of instrument, 26
  angles, 28
Sharpening of instruments, 165-174
Shepherd's hook explorer, 4
Shilder plugger, 88
Sickle scaler, 122-123
Sickles
  sharpening, 172-174
  surgical, 101
Silicon carbide abrasive, 47
Silver cones, 86
Silver point pliers, 86
Simple articulator, 10
Slabs, mixing, 8
Snap head mandrels, 50
Snap-on head prophylaxis angle, 131
Soft-tissue surgical instruments, 136-142
Spatulas, 9
Spoon excavator, 38
  long-shank, 69
Spoon-shaped cotton roll holders, 21
Spreader(s)
  D-11 and no. 3 endodontic, 87

Spreader(s)—cont'd
    finger, 89
Standard bevel chisel, 29
Starlite rubber dam frame, 76
Stationary instrument and moving stone technique, 172
Stationary stone and moving instrument technique, 173
Steam heat sterilization, 176
Sterilization of instruments, 175-181
Stone(s), 47
    mounted rotary, 167
    moving, and stationary instrument technique, 172
    sharpening, 166
        care of, 174
    stationary, and moving instrument technique, 173
    unmounted, 167
Straight angle shank, 28
Straight bur, 43
Straight chisels, 30
Straight elevator, 150
Straight handpiece mandrel
    extra-long, 50
    pinhead screw, 50
    screw, 50
    snap, 50
Straight handpieces, 40
Straight scissors, 19
Strap rubber dam frame, 14
Strips, polishing, 135
Surgery, endodontic periapical, instruments, 91-92
Surgical burs, 91, 161
Surgical instruments, periodontal, 136-145
Surgical mallet, 160
Surgical scissors, 162
Svedopter, 80
Svedopter saliva ejector, 22-23
Sweeney handle, 52, 53
Syringe
    endodontic irrigating, 75
    Luer-Lok, 75

T

Tape, dental, 134
T-bar elevator, 152
Thumb forceps, 6
Tofflemire retainers, 56
Torquing key, 96
Towel clamp, Bachus, 12
Trays, orthodontic impression, 109
Trimmers, gingival margin, 36-37
Triple shank, 28
Triple-angle chisels, 33
Triple-beaked pliers, 99
Tweed arch-adjusting pliers, 93
Tweed loop-forming pliers, 116

U

U-shaped rubber dam frame, 14
Ultrasonic cleaner, 175
Ultrasonic scaling device, 130
Universal maxillary forceps, 153
Unmounted stones, 167
Utility pliers
    Howe, 103
    Weingart, 115

V

Vacuum-ejector system, 24-25

W

Wafer, absorbent, 21
Weingart utility pliers, 115
Wheel finishing burs, 45
Wheels, 49
White, S.S., and dental history, 2
White stones, 47
Whittler, Neivert, 167
Woodson no. 2 plastic endodontic instrument, 72

Y

Young rubber dam frame, 76